The
Fibromyalgia
Solution

The
Fibromyalgia
Solution

*A Breakthrough Approach
to Heal Your Body and
Take Back Your Life*

David Dryland, MD
with Lorie List

**WELLNESS
CENTRAL**

NEW YORK   BOSTON

Copyright © 2004, 2007 by David Dryland, MD

All rights reserved. Except as permitted under the U.S. Copyright Act of 1976, no part of this publication may be reproduced, distributed, or transmitted in any form or by any means, or stored in a database or retrieval system, without the prior written permission of the publisher.

Wellness Central
Hachette Book Group USA
237 Park Avenue
New York, NY 10017

Visit our Web site at www.HachetteBookGroupUSA.com.

Printed in the United States of America
First Edition: May 2007

10 9 8 7 6 5 4 3 2

Wellness Central is an imprint of Grand Central Publishing.
The Wellness Central name and logo is a trademark of Hachette Book Group USA, Inc.

Library of Congress Cataloging-in-Publication Data
Dryland, David.
The fibromyalgia solution: a breakthrough approach to heal your body and take back your life / David Dryland, with Lorie C. List.—1st ed.
p. cm.
Includes bibliographical references and index.
Summary: "A new treatment by a leading rheumatologist, featuring the little-known off-label use of a widely available medication, for the millions of Americans suffering from fibromyalgia."
—Provided by the publisher.
ISBN 978-0-446-69817-7
1. Fibromyalgia—Popular works. I. List, Lorie C. II. Title.
RC927.3.D79 2007
616.7' 42—dc22   2006022837

For fibromyalgia patients everywhere.

Acknowledgments

Many people helped make this book possible. First and foremost, I'd like to thank all my fibromyalgia patients who showed tremendous courage in the face of adversity and were willing to find a last reservoir of hope when it seemed none existed. Without their willingness to once again take up the fight against something they believed was a lost cause, the material for this book would still be ideas in my head. Thanks to them, we now know that recovery from fibromyalgia is not a fluke or an accident but a deliberate, step-by-step process that anyone can undertake. Tremendous thanks go to Cherie Taylor for all her support, hard work, and belief in this project. Thanks to Austin VanKampen and Laney D'Aquino for the illustrations. I am also grateful to Mark Scarpaci of Ashland Creative for his help with the earliest phases of this process.

I'd also like to thank my agent, Stephanie Tade, for seeing the promise of this book and finding a home for it with Hachette Book Group. Much appreciation goes to my editor, Natalie Kaire, who did a superb job of shepherding this project through the many different stages of book writing. Thanks also to Daric Lucero of Ashland Community Hospital Physical Therapy for providing helpful insights regarding exercise for fibromyalgia patients. The advice of the clinical nutritionist Kia Sanford of Kailo Counseling was invaluable in putting together information on nutrition and diet.

Finally, a word of acknowledgment is in order for all the medical researchers noted in this book. Without their tireless quest for knowledge, we would still be operating off assumptions and best guesses regarding the cause of fibromyalgia.

Contents

Foreword

No one sets out to be a fibromyalgia specialist.

Those of us in healthcare choose to participate in patient care for a variety of reasons, but not everyone has the stamina and desire to tackle our most daunting medical disorders. Physicians can make significant contributions to science, to the health and well-being of their patients, and to career fulfillment but still not engage in the daily stress of trying to cure the untreatable. Historically, treating fibromyalgia patients has not been for everyone.

But, on occasion, there are physicians and other caregivers who rise above to fight the losing battle and support the less popular and forgotten. Many physicians still hope that fibromyalgia will simply go away so they can get back to "real medicine." Others remain skeptical of its very existence despite the millions of Americans afflicted. A smaller group, for reasons of their own, choose the road less traveled—a road that may someday lead to a cure for fibromyalgia. David Dryland, MD, has chosen such a path and has demonstrated his conviction to this cause by sharing his views with you in *The Fibromyalgia Solution*.

I first met David at an informal Sunday-morning breakfast at a medical conference in 2001. While discussing research relating to the use of new medications for the treatment of fibromyalgia, I mentioned that my life as a physician was "getting easier." New medications used to reduce an over-active stress, or fight-or-flight, response in the brain were improving sleep quality and decreasing pain for patients with fibromyalgia. Prior to these discoveries, my office life had been a misery, since I had very little to offer these patients. During every stressful holiday or Pacific storm, my staff and I would be overwhelmed by phone calls from desperate patients with fibromyalgia. Their symptoms had flared up in response to the stress, and I was unable to help them.

Stress is a fundamental concern for all living beings, but its effect physiologically is to prompt an appropriate response. The stress of fearing a tiger prompts us to flee. If cornered by a tiger, we fight with a monumental adrenaline (epinephrine) surge. But this system, better known to physicians as the auto-nomic nervous system (ANS), must be balanced and working properly to maintain good physical and emotional health. Over-activity of the stress response ruins sleep quality and wreaks havoc on many other basic housekeeping functions that are also controlled by the ANS, including the regulation of normal bowel, bladder, cardiac, immune, metabolic, and temperature status. Many of these systems appear to have a mind of their own in patients with fibromyalgia, so understanding how stress works can lead to understanding many of these other problems as well.

As this stress response began to be understood and addressed with the new medications, fibromyalgia pain and fatigue in my patients began to wane. Eventually, a few patients actu-ally recovered completely. This was the break needed for us to begin to sort out the puzzle of fibromyalgia. I have often told patients that, as clinicians, we are interested in why you hurt, but we are much more interested in why you are better. If we understand what made you better, we may understand what needs to be done to solve your problem completely.

Fundamentally, for those who had recovered, their stress response had changed. Their hair trigger for an excessive stress and arousal response had become more balanced and appropriate. These recovered patients finally slept normally. Previously, some patients might have improved but were rarely symptom-free. These completely symptom-free patients represented a true breakthrough in understanding fibromyalgia.

For those still suffering with only a list of medication side effects to show for their efforts, it can be disconcerting to even imagine that other patients have already completely recovered from fibromyalgia. But it is true. Dr. Dryland confirmed these observations in his own patients and then took the next important step to thoroughly consider many additional treatment approaches that could work just as well, without the use of medications.

About the same time as my conversations with him took place in 2001, animal models of stress and basic research on central neurotransmitters, especially dopamine, had uncovered a major piece of the fibromyalgia puzzle. A new approach to understanding fibromyalgia emerged that considered dopamine and its role as a regulator of those basic housekeeping functions already mentioned, including sleep, temperature regulation, bowel motility, stomach acid production, metabolic rate, immunity, heart rate, blood pressure, bladder function, and the fight-or-flight response. It was becoming increasingly clear that all these functions, including the stress response, were controlled by the ANS and regulated by dopamine. Supportive of this concept, all of these other body functions improved simultaneously as these first few people who took the new medications completely recovered from fibromyalgia.

Until these discoveries, fibromyalgia was the ultimate mystery. But for those who investigate medical puzzles, there remains a basic tenet: no matter what the problem, there is always a cause. It is just a matter of whether we are smart enough to find it. The ANS is the final frontier of medicine. Despite being just as important as the heart, liver, or immune system, it is poorly understood and often ignored. When working properly, this system protects us in many ways. But when its activity fluctuates widely, as it does in patients with fibromyalgia, a remarkably complex array of problems can occur. Through the following chapters, you will begin to understand its importance to your health, how it fails, and how to restore its normal function.

It will not be long before we have the proper tools to measure the fundamental biochemistry of stress. In the meantime, Dr. Dryland has provided a guide outlining many important concepts and treatment options to effectively rebalance the abnormal stress response driving fibromyalgia. It will take some time for these new concepts to be digested by the medical world at large, but this is a very exciting and significant time for those with fibromyalgia.

Eventually, understanding the ANS will change how physicians treat patients forever. Clinicians will consider all medical disorders, not just fibromyalgia, in the context of autonomic regulation. Just as blood pressure, heart rate, temperature, and weight are assessed at clinic visits, autonomic activity will eventually become part of these basic tests. In the future, clinicians will look back and remember that teasing apart the nuances of the ANS in an effort to help patients with fibromyalgia was the beginning of it all.

It almost seems too good to be true, but I am reminded by patients daily of how far we have come. As patients with fibromyalgia realize, everyone seems to have a miracle cure these days. What is uncommon is to receive guidance from someone with scientific qualifications, rheumatology training, and exceptional insight who is also immersed in the role of treating patients on a daily basis, like Dr. Dryland. He has approached fibromyalgia comprehensively, with an emphasis on positive intervention and the restoration of good health. His recommendations for addressing fibromyalgia are based on the best scientific research available, combined with excellent intuitive reasoning and extensive clinical experience.

When books like *The Fibromyalgia Solution* are finally written, one often wonders why someone did not have these insights before. But that is the measure of true knowledge. Every important discovery or basic truth seems so simple in retrospect. Dr. Dryland has a right to be proud of his achievements, something I know he hears from his own patients already. His approach truly helps patients with fibromyalgia recover.

The human element of fibromyalgia extends beyond patients to include their caregivers. Clinicians need to take more interest in fibromyalgia, but sometimes our technocentric training gets in the way. I always teach the internal medicine residents and medical students that their primary resource is courage. Courage provides the strength to persevere, to empathize, and to care for patients, even when we fear failure. It also takes courage to consider new ideas like the ones presented in this book. Thankfully, Dr. Dryland can be counted among those who embraced courage and continued to search for answers to the epic challenge of fibromyalgia.

Andrew J. Holman, MD
Assistant Clinical Professor of Medicine
University of Washington
Pacific Rheumatology Associates

Introduction

Fibromyalgia is one of the most devastating and misunderstood illnesses of our time. If you have fibromyalgia, you know exactly what I am talking about. You understand the unending pain and relentless fatigue firsthand. You know what it's like to wake up day after day feeling exhausted and in pain and yet still be expected to function. You know the frustration of not being believed and being told that there's nothing wrong with you. Even when people believe you, they can't really understand all the ways in which your world has fallen apart. If you have fibromyalgia, you want answers to these basic questions: Why did this happen to me? How can I be in so much pain all the time? Why am I so exhausted? Why is there always something else wrong with my body? What can I do to get better?

No matter how much research you've done, I'm sure you haven't found the answers you want. Most doctors, books, articles, and Web sites on fibromyalgia offer you little hope for either understanding why you developed this painful and debilitating condition or, more important, how you can get better. Instead, they describe different ways to manage your symptoms and how to live with the pain. The first paragraph of virtually anything you read about fibromyalgia still explains that the causes are not fully understood and that there is no known cure.

As a result, no one will tell you that you can recover. But they should, because you can.

The belief that fibromyalgia is incurable is so deeply ingrained in the dogma of mainstream medicine that almost everyone has failed to realize that science has already provided the answers most people are still looking for. What you are about to read will change everything you thought you knew about fibromyalgia. Whether this is the first book you've read on fibromyalgia or the tenth, it will be the last one you will ever need. Most books on fibromyalgia are about how to live with this supposedly incurable condition. They are essentially survival guides that recommend a dizzying array of options that may or may not help you feel better. This book is not about survival, it's about solutions! Far more than simply describing the questions that surround fibromyalgia, this book provides the answers that you want now! When you've finished reading this book, you'll not only understand why you have fibromyalgia, you'll also understand the path to recovery. If you follow my advice and stick to the program outlined in this book, you'll find that it is within your power to take control of your health and your life. I am not making empty promises. I am offering a solution grounded in science and backed by my own personal research and the research of other experts in their respective fields of science. It's also based on my own experience as a former fibromyalgia sufferer and my daily work as a physician treating people just like you.

When I decided to specialize in rheumatology, I knew that I would be helping people in a great deal of physical pain. Rheumatologists help people who suffer from very painful and chronic illnesses such as rheumatoid arthritis, osteoarthritis, lupus, and fibromyalgia. I didn't realize that I would be largely unprepared to help over 20 percent of my patients, basically anyone suffering from fibromyalgia. Although many people have never heard of fibromyalgia, it is actually the second most common disorder seen by rheumatologists. It is more common than rheumatoid arthritis and easily as disabling. Fibromyalgia accounts for 20 to 25 percent of the patients seen by rheumatologists—a figure that is even more startling when you consider that there are about one hundred fibromyalgia sufferers for every twenty who make it to a rheumatologist. I quickly realized that fibromyalgia is a very lonely and almost invisible illness suffered by an astonishing number of people.

I didn't learn much about fibromyalgia in medical school, mostly because there wasn't a lot of information about what caused it or how to help people who suffer from it. In fact, a lot of my professors didn't even believe it was a legitimate medical diagnosis. They saw it as something that belonged in the realm of psychology, assuming that the pain was simply all in a patient's head. Those professors didn't believe in fibromyalgia because they couldn't find any tangible evidence that something was wrong. As a new doctor, fresh from my rheumatology fellowship at Yale University, I was extremely frustrated with my inability to provide my fibromyalgia patients with help of any real consequence for their condition. My frustration, however, paled in comparison to theirs. They wanted answers, and I didn't have any. At the time, I never imagined that in order to find answers, I would first have to face my own battle with fibromyalgia.

When I was diagnosed with fibromyalgia myself, I felt frustrated, helpless, and completely confounded by the unnerving and unrelenting symptoms I experienced. At the time, no one, including my fellow rheumatologists, could help me. I turned to my medical textbooks and other popular books on fibromyalgia for more information. The books I read on fibromyalgia fell into three categories. The first category of books I found presented an already old school notion that fibromyalgia was some form of arthritis in the muscles. It is now widely accepted that although muscle pain is common in fibromyalgia, the muscles are not actually to blame. A second category of books offered inadequately supported theories, false promises, and lopsided advice for people looking for anything that might help. The third category of books on fibromyalgia offered a more well-rounded picture of the illness and practical advice on how to manage the symptoms. In recent years, this third category of books has begun to more accurately describe fibromyalgia as a central sensitization problem. The premise behind central sensitization is that problems within the central nervous system (CNS) cause you to become hypersensitive to all of your sensations. These books describe some of the latest research on different chemical imbalances seen in fibromyalgia sufferers and offer reasonable guesses as to why these imbalances cause some of your symptoms. They do not, however, explain the true causes of fibromyalgia or provide information on how to restore balance to your CNS and recover. This book does.

I have developed a completely new approach to the diagnosis and treatment of fibromyalgia. I do much more than treat the symptoms of fibromyalgia—I show people how to resolve the underlying causes. Fibromyalgia is not a disease. It stems from a processing problem in the CNS that amplifies any type of stimulus received by your body. People without fibromyalgia have a natural filter that blocks out, or at least tunes down, a lot of the signals initially picked up by the CNS. Imagine taking off this filter and instead attaching a megaphone to the part of your nervous system that processes messages and sends them to the brain. That's fibromyalgia. Although these amplified signals clearly cause you a lot of misery, they don't permanently harm your body. One of the most important breakthroughs described in this book is the identification of the exact chemical responsible for this processing breakdown in the CNS. By far, the most important imbalance is the depletion of dopamine. Dopamine is the chemical that normally helps filter your sensations. A lack of dopamine leads to the hypersensitivity and pain that characterize fibromyalgia. Once I understood the physiological cause of fibromyalgia, I was able to cure it by teaching patients how to rebuild their dopamine reserves, restoring the balance of their CNS and enabling them to move past fibromyalgia.

I never imagined writing a book on fibromyalgia. I'll be the first to admit that I'm a doctor, not necessarily a writer. However, as I began having more and more success in helping people recover, I knew that I had to find a way to take this knowledge outside the walls of my clinical practice. Helping people recover from fibromyalgia is more involved than a twenty-minute office visit. At the request of my patients and the local medical community, I began leading workshops and seminars designed to educate healthcare providers and patients alike about the true causes of fibromyalgia and how to recover. As I traveled from city to city, simple word-of-mouth advertising and public-service announcements drew hundreds of people to my seminars. Many of these people could not find a specialist who would accept them as a patient once they were diagnosed with fibromyalgia. My explanation of fibromyalgia and documented success stories of patients who had recovered came as a complete shock to people who had previously been told that nothing could be done for their suffering. My goal at those seminars was always to provide all the information people needed to recover. However, it's a lot of information to digest in one sitting, and people always left full of hope and gratitude but wanting more information. This book evolved from those experiences, in combination with my hands-on treatment of patients in my office.

In my office, I work with each patient to develop an individualized treatment plan that meets his or her specific needs. Each of these treatment plans fits within the framework of a standardized program anyone can follow, and this is the program on which this book is based. Every case of fibromyalgia is different. But in every case, there is a predictable sequence of steps that led to the manifestation of this condition. I'll show you how to trace those steps and then start working backward in order to rebalance your CNS. If you follow the program outlined in this book, you'll be able to develop an individualized recovery plan in much the same way as a patient who comes to my office. This book will help you unlock the secrets of fibromyalgia and put the key to recovery into your hands.

I have divided the information in *The Fibromyalgia Solution* into two parts. Part 1 demystifies fibromyalgia, explaining its causes and how they lead to your symptoms. I will show you how I discovered the true cause of fibromyalgia. I will also help you determine whether you have fibromyalgia or another condition that might be causing your symptoms. In recent years, there has been a flood of new information regarding fibromyalgia. I will help you put the latest information in the context of your own body and teach you how to use this information to recover your health.

In part 2, you will learn how to develop your own individualized program for recovery. I highly recommend finding a physician, nurse practitioner, or other qualified healthcare professional to help you follow this program. Part 2 will teach you how to feel better immediately so that you have the strength you need to follow your program. You will learn about different medications and natural supplements that can help with symptoms and how to resolve the sleep problems and effectively manage the stress and anxiety that are common in fibromyalgia patients. I will discuss dietary changes that can make a world of difference, an exercise program that's right for your body, and complementary therapies that have a solid track record of helping people with fibromyalgia feel better. You will also find a detailed discussion of a class of drugs that virtually eliminate all symptoms of fibromyalgia. Most important, you will learn how to reverse the course of fibromyalgia and begin reclaiming your life. At the end of the book, I've included a list of additional books and online resources that you will find helpful in your journey.

If you have fibromyalgia, it is important to keep in mind that you did not develop it overnight, and neither will you recover overnight. However, if you follow my program, it is likely that your overall health will improve in a short period of time, giving you the strength and stamina to finish the program and take back your life.

My goal in writing this book is to empower people to help themselves as much as possible, regardless of how the health-care community decides to respond to this growing crisis. So far, the biggest reaction to the increased fibromyalgia population has come from people seeking to make a profit off those who are desperate enough to entertain any offhand promise of relief, once they are given a life sentence of pain and suffering. There are many products out there that might help you feel better by relieving some of your symptoms. The important thing to remember is that none of these products will provide lasting relief, no matter what they promise.

The true, secret ingredient to recovering your health is knowledge. Information is power. It is your weapon in what is likely the most difficult battle you have ever faced. The remarkable thing about fibromyalgia is that once you understand how this illness works, you have the power to heal from within. It doesn't necessarily take a lot of expensive trips to the doctor or supplements with ingredients you've never heard of. What it does take is courage in the face of adversity, inner strength in the midst of outer weakness, and a desire to take your life back that outweighs the obstacles you may encounter.

If you successfully follow the program outlined in this book, you can join the ranks of those who have recovered from fibromyalgia. These are people who had all but given up any hope of getting better until they came to my office or attended one of my seminars. And they didn't just get better, they left fibromyalgia behind forever. The comprehensive nature of the program outlined in this book will likely challenge you on physical, emotional, and intellectual levels. That's because the goal of my program is to help you completely reverse the fibromyalgia cycle until you are fully free of its grasp. Once you have reached that goal, you will once again be free to enjoy life as you please, without ever worrying about the repercussions of a fibromyalgia flare. You simply won't have fibromyalgia anymore.

The most important step you can take right now is to believe that your body can heal. The path to recovery is not always easy, but it is filled with large and small rewards along the way as you reclaim pieces of yourself and your life that you had resigned to memories. Fibromyalgia is a tremendously hard journey and not one I would wish on anyone. However, as is true with most of life's challenges, there is a silver lining to the pain and suffering in your life. With recovery comes a deep and lasting appreciation of all the joy and beauty each new day has to offer. I wish you the best as you take your first steps down the path to recovery.

PART I

Understanding Fibromyalgia

CHAPTER 1

The Frustration of Fibromyalgia

Sophie's Story

Sophie, a successful young woman in her early thirties, had been sick for almost a year by the time she first came to my office. Her world was rapidly unraveling, and neither she nor anyone else could figure out why. When I walked into the exam room, she handed me a comprehensive chart of everything that had happened in her life over the past sixteen months. She had painstakingly pieced together a record, month by month, listing the symptoms she had experienced, the doctors she had seen, the treatments she had sought, and the medications she had taken. She also included her activity level as well as an overview of events in both her work and personal life. She put the chart together because she just couldn't make sense of her complex symptoms: their variety, when they occurred, or why they got worse. She instinctively knew that somehow all of her diverse and seemingly unrelated physical ailments *had* to be linked to one another. She hoped I could tell her how.

I looked at her chart. Before pain and illness invaded her body, it seemed as though Sophie enjoyed a great life. She owned a house, had a good job, and lived in a beautiful area. On any given weekend, depending on the season, you might find her exploring the mountains on horseback, running white water in her kayak, skiing with friends, hiking up a new trail, or camping under the stars. I scanned her chart carefully, noting that as her symptoms increased, her activity level steadily decreased.

Sophie explained to me that she had pain just about everywhere. Like many other fibromyalgia patients, Sophie woke up every morning feeling as though she was in a train wreck the night before. After lying on her aching muscles all night, her bed felt like a slab of concrete, and she felt too tired to get up but too uncomfortable not to. She suffered frequent neck spasms, her ribs hurt when she took a deep breath, her back hurt if she sat for more than a few moments, and her arms and wrists ached as if she had been beaten with a steel bat. It hurt for Sophie to grip or even lift the smallest of everyday tools, such as a pen or coffee mug. She couldn't drive, feed her horses, hold hands with her husband, or even scratch her dog on the head. She had to drink everything out of a straw because lifting a glass full of liquid was out of the question. She had made her living as a writer but could no longer bear the pain of sitting at a computer for hours at a time.

In addition to her constant pain, Sophie felt sick all the time. Her allergies had been overwhelming that year. She had never had asthma before, but this past summer she could hardly walk up a hill without having an asthma attack. She felt like she had a never-ending case of the flu and collapsed by 2 p.m. every day. After 2 p.m. she watched the clock, waiting for it to be late enough to go to bed. On better days she would take a short walk, but any other activity was out of the question. Walking even made her *arms* hurt more. That was the thing, she said. Everything hurt so much more than it should. She had tried to ski once that winter, but when she fell on her hip, it hurt intensely for a week instead of just being bruised and sore for a day or two. She became afraid of taking part in any activity in which she might risk a fall or injury.

When Sophie came to see me, she had already seen fourteen healthcare providers, including one in an emergency room. She had tried well over a dozen different medications for sleep, pain, and possible infections. There were X-rays, an MRI scan, an extremely painful nerve-conduction test, painful trigger-point injections, and a comprehensive set of blood work to test for possible conditions and diseases. Nothing explained the pain and illness that Sophie couldn't shake.

Each doctor's visit was an emotional roller coaster. She wanted answers desperately, but she didn't want to find out that she had lupus, carpal tunnel syndrome, nerve problems, rheumatoid arthritis, Lyme disease, or any of the other things she was being tested for. When tests came back negative, she felt relief but also anguish that she still didn't know what was wrong. She, too, felt a bit like she was starting to lose her mind. With so much pain, how come nobody could find something wrong with her? Two of her doctors halfheartedly whispered the word "fibromyalgia," but one specifically said he didn't want to give her that label.

Fibromyalgia was the one answer Sophie knew she didn't want. She had done her research, and every time she read about fibromyalgia, the symptoms sounded all too familiar. The problem she saw with fibromyalgia was that doctors didn't really know what it was, and according to every Web site she looked at, people with fibromyalgia didn't get better. It seemed like a last-resort diagnosis, and that wasn't what she wanted.

She didn't want to "learn to live with the symptoms," which is the prognosis most fibromyalgia patients receive. She wanted to know how to get better. She couldn't bear the thought of moving through life in such a slow, painful way—one in which time was measured in pain-filled moments rather than joy-filled hours or days. One of her deepest fears was that the pain would prevent her from having children.

Does Sophie's story sound all too familiar? Chances are, you're reading this book because either you or someone you love struggles with fibromyalgia. Can you relate to the patients who come into my office and tell me they feel like their lives are literally collapsing? They are women and men who, until their bodies were assaulted with endless pain, fatigue, and other inexplicable symptoms, were healthy, active people who were either enjoying their lives or at least making the most of what life had to offer them. As a whole, my patients are ambitious, driven, hard workers who care deeply about leading a meaningful life. Many of them were previously diagnosed with fibromyalgia and told that the best modern medicine might offer is help with some of the symptoms. If you've heard a similar story in your search for answers, don't believe it. Fibromyalgia is no longer a dead-end diagnosis.

Fibromyalgia Symptoms

Fibromyalgia feels different to everyone. The common denominator in most cases is an elevated awareness of painful and uncomfortable sensations throughout the body. The pain can be diffuse or localized, and it can move from one part of the body to another. Most patients complain of pain and stiffness in their neck and shoulders or in other stiff, tight muscles. For a lot of people, there is general tenderness throughout the body. Painful sensations may be described as aching, burning, or throbbing. What hurt intensely yesterday may only be a mild ache today. In fact, so many places can hurt that at a doctor's visit, a patient may only focus on the things that really hurt that day. Confounding to doctor and patient, such an account distorts the picture of the illness and often prevents an accurate diagnosis from being made.

Fibromyalgia patients are chronically tired and often wake up feeling as if they didn't sleep at all. Depression is common, but who wouldn't get depressed by unending, unexplained misery? Many people experience memory, concentration, and cognition problems—a condition commonly known as fibro fog. Fibro fog is actually one of the more frustrating symptoms people experience, making it difficult to multitask, concentrate at work, or think on their feet. Other symptoms include headaches, numbness, skin irritation, feeling too cold or too hot, sensitivity to bright lights or loud noises, and an aversion to intense tastes and smells. Due to a depressed immune system, fibromyalgia patients are more likely to catch a cold. They will be sick longer and have a longer recovery period. Existing or previously undetected allergies can become unbearable. Many fibromyalgia patients also suffer from irritable bowel syndrome, adding tremendously to their discomfort.

Headaches and heartaches go hand in hand with fibromyalgia, as you struggle to maintain relationships, jobs, and even simple daily routines. Fibromyalgia symptoms can come and go, leaving you enormously frustrated with your inability to know how you will feel on any given day. Adding insult to injury is the fact that no matter how terrible you feel, you can still appear healthy to everyone else. An initial outpouring of sympathy from friends and family will often fade as the illness drags on without any explanation. Physicians have trouble identifying a physical cause that explains the continued pain.

Common Fibromyalgia Symptoms

- widespread, variable aches and pains
- fatigue
- morning stiffness
- restless sleep
- pain exacerbated by exercise
- noninflammatory pain that doesn't respond to medication
- increased sensitivity to allergens
- confusion or difficulty concentrating
- headaches
- abdominal cramping
- numbness or tingling
- easily irritated skin
- sensitivity to temperature
- sensitivity to bright lights or loud noises
- sensitivity to intense tastes or smells
- skin that readily flushes
- discomfort in crowds

Even when a physical cause is identified, such as a strained back, the pain is always far greater than would be expected for the type of injury.

Fibromyalgia is full of cruel ironies. It makes you too tired to get out of bed, while at the same time, lying on a mattress is so unbearable, you can't stand to stay there. You will want nothing more than to fall into a deep sleep but find yourself staring at the clock instead. Exercise that feels great one day leaves you in agony the next day. You won't feel like drinking, but you'll still feel like you have a hangover. And on the day when you wake up knowing you would do anything to get your health back, you are too exhausted to figure out how on your own.

A Brief History of Fibromyalgia

For decades, fibromyalgia patients have struggled in silence, as much of the medical world turned a blind eye to their plight. It was less than twenty-five years ago that modern medicine officially recognized fibromyalgia as a clinical diagnosis. People have suffered from it for much longer. Hippocrates first described a similar set of symptoms in 400 BC. Not until 1816 did the British surgeon William Balfour once again make note of the condition. In 1904, the British physician Sir William Gowers classified this set of symptoms as fibrositis, now known as fibromyalgia, indicating a medical condition that stemmed from inflammation of the muscles. Fibromyalgia was considered "arthritis of the muscles" and classified with other rheumatological conditions involving pain in the muscles or joints. (Rheumatological conditions are a set of diseases generally involving inflammation of joints or other tissues, such as gout or rheumatoid arthritis.) Early research did indicate slight abnormalities in the muscles of fibromyalgia patients, but these theories were later disproved. Once it became clear that there was no inflammation in the muscles, there was no longer any logical explanation as to why fibromyalgia caused pain.

Throughout most of the last century, many physicians thought of fibromyalgia as a purely psychosomatic condition, and in the beginning that was an understandable reaction. Their patients complained of pain in their muscles and joints despite the fact that the physicians couldn't find anything wrong. Until the 1990s, there were no guidelines on how to diagnose fibromyalgia, and most physicians dismissed the condition or made the diagnosis by default when they couldn't find anything else responsible for the pain.

As early as 1981, the fibromyalgia research pioneer Dr. Muhammad Yunnus conducted clinical studies of patients with fibromyalgia and identified a wider range of symptoms than the muscle pain that commonly occurred in these patients. He was one of the first researchers to understand that the symptoms these patients experienced were not only real but somehow interconnected. He called for physicians to base a fibromyalgia diagnosis on its own characteristic features rather than on the absence of another recognizable condition. Sadly, this advice fell on deaf ears, and fibromyalgia continued to be thought of as the diagnosis doctors used when they failed to find another problem. In many cases, this is still true today.

Eventually, the population of fibromyalgia patients became too big to simply ignore. In 1987, the American Medical Association (AMA) finally recognized fibromyalgia as an illness and cause of disability. The American College of Rheumatology (ACR) followed suit in 1990, establishing much-needed "official" diagnostic criteria. While the newfound recognition and specific diagnostic criteria certainly helped validate fibromyalgia's existence as a clinical disorder, it didn't help answer any questions about the nature of the illness or why some people got it when others didn't. Furthermore, the name still referred to the old belief that the problem was primarily in the muscles. *Fibro* means fibrous (as in muscle fibers), *myo* means muscle, and *algia* means pain—*muscle fiber pain*. Despite the fact that these changes didn't actually answer the important questions about fibromyalgia, they still helped a lot of people simply by validating their suffering. Researchers have found that people with fibromyalgia actually feel better about themselves and their condition once they have a diagnosis, even though that diagnosis has not traditionally offered any tangible relief. There is, however, tremendous mental relief in being able to put a name to your illness.

A Daunting Medical Challenge

Since fibromyalgia was officially recognized, it has been one of medicine's most confounding disorders. Symptoms are highly varied and can come and go intermittently, making it extremely frustrating to diagnose. Unfortunately, most doctors are trained to treat existing and known conditions, and very few have the time to take on the unexplainable in a twenty-minute office visit. As a result, fibromyalgia patients go from doctor to doctor, hoping for answers. Typical fibromyalgia patients visit one doctor per month and wind up in the hospital once every three years. They have a high incidence of surgeries and a disproportionately high occurrence of carpal tunnel syndrome and other pain-related problems. Surgeries are rarely successful and can sometimes make their suffering even worse. Many are misdiagnosed and may even undergo unnecessary surgery. The average fibromyalgia patient suffers for five years or more and sees between five and fifteen doctors before receiving an accurate diagnosis. Even when people are finally diagnosed, they have a label, which is more than they had before, but not nearly enough.

The ACR conservatively estimates that up to six million people in the United States have fibromyalgia. That's about one person in fifty. Other organizations and experts estimate that eight to ten million people suffer from fibromyalgia—one in thirty-four. Personally, I believe that about one out of ten people is suffering from fibromyalgia, having either the preliminary stages or the full-blown disorder. Consider the fact that at any given time, 10 to 12 percent of the population reports chronic, generalized pain unrelated to a structural or inflammatory cause. That percentage represents thirty million people in this country who may have fibromyalgia or are seriously at risk of developing this disabling condition. A lot of these people gradually get better, and that constant ache becomes a distant memory. However, just because they get better doesn't mean they didn't have a brush with fibromyalgia. These patients may have sought treatment, but their symptoms, being relatively less severe, allowed rest, pain alleviation, and self-nurturing to facilitate natural remission. It was not necessary for their condition to be exhaustively explored or for any official diagnosis to be made. These statistics paint an important picture of a common and devastating illness that has been shunned by modern medicine. More important is that behind each one of these statistics is a real person whose life has been torn apart by pain, confusion, and unending frustration.

Perhaps it is due to the long-standing dominance of men in medicine that fibromyalgia patients struggled so hard for recognition. Approximately 85 percent of fibromyalgia patients are female. Back in the 1970s and 1980s, when increasing numbers of women were complaining of fibromyalgia symptoms, more than 80 percent of physicians were men. Too many of those male physicians of past generations simply couldn't relate to women complaining of pain not immediately traceable to an obvious medical condition. Men have also suffered from the long-standing view of fibromyalgia as a "female illness." As a result, men are much less likely to be correctly diagnosed with fibromyalgia or to even have it considered as a possible problem.

Although attitudes about fibromyalgia have shifted radically in the past decade, there remains an undercurrent of mistrust and suspicion regarding this illness that runs through the medical community. As I have traveled, leading seminars on fibromyalgia, I have encountered entire cities where not a single rheumatologist will accept fibromyalgia patients. A national shortage of rheumatologists combined with an aging population means that patients suffering from even the most serious cases of arthritis may have to wait as long as seven months to see a rheumatologist. As a consequence, too many rheumatologists believe that they should reserve their time for those patients with diseases they can understand and help treat through a proven medical regimen. The implications of this situation are profound not only for patients and doctors but also for those responsible for setting healthcare policies. The growing number of untreated fibromyalgia cases causes more suffering, more disabilities, and more insurance claims than ever before. Consider that 26 percent of people with fibromyalgia report receiving some type of disability payment. Close to 30 percent of patients report difficulty maintaining a job. When calculated in terms of medical fees, lost wages, diminished work productivity, disability benefits, and other societal expenses, the costs of fibromyalgia likely exceed ten billion dollars per year.

The Slow Pace of Research

The amount of research being done on fibromyalgia has increased exponentially over the past decade. This surge of research was greatly aided by the establishment of diagnostic criteria in 1990. Once the diagnostic criteria was established and fibromyalgia gained traction as a legitimate illness, research began in earnest. However, with such a complicated illness, it can take a lot of small discoveries in seemingly unrelated areas of medicine to add up to any useful answers. Even though advances in science continually change the face of medicine, change can happen at a snail's pace. For someone waiting for an answer to pain, the pace of research moves on a geologic timescale. Scientists develop hypotheses, write grant proposals, get funding (if they're lucky), painstakingly set up their studies, patiently cultivate their petri dishes, and hopefully come up with something groundbreaking along the way. Then, the results of the research are discussed, written about, and submitted to medical journals for eventual publication. Other scientists read about the results, develop their own hypotheses, and slowly repeat the same process. Scientific discoveries rarely come in a sudden flash of luck, genius, or something in between—although that certainly does happen. Instead, they are pieced together, one small discovery at a time. When the public hears about the "latest medical development," chances are that particular development has been simmering in laboratories and medical journals for a decade or more.

In recent years, a steady stream of credible medical research shedding new light on fibromyalgia has begun to appear in the pages of medical journals, some of which even seeps into the mainstream media. But that information is helpful only when it is pieced together in a way that helps patients understand their condition and learn how to recover. Even as new discoveries help shed light on the problem, doctors often hesitate to apply this new information in their practices until the treatment becomes mainstream. Unfortunately for fibromyalgia patients, this reluctance to share new information leaves a lot of desperate people in the dark.

CHAPTER 2

Making Sense of Fibromyalgia

Every night, it was the same. Lying in bed, my body felt like it was on fire. At times, I thought I would go out of my mind with the urge to scratch my arms and legs. Instead of sleeping, I would find myself in the bathroom applying cream to my intensely painful skin. The prescription cream, guaranteed by my dermatologist to relieve any rash, was utterly useless on mine. Covered in balm, I would return to bed and try to sleep. Sometimes, my skin would feel comfortable enough that I would just start to drift off. Then, just before the refuge of sleep, my body would jerk awake. As the minutes on my alarm clock clicked by, the horrible itchiness would return in full force. Soon, I'd start worrying about not getting enough sleep. Before long, I'd trudge back to the bathroom to put on more skin cream, and the whole cycle would start over again. This could go on all night. Knowing that I had to see patients in the morning, I would take a sleeping pill and finally drift off in the last hours before dawn.

That's how my symptoms started, with an inexplicable and painful itching. I wondered what was happening to me. Even when I wasn't going crazy feeling too hot or itchy, I couldn't sleep. My mind was always racing, planning, and worrying. I replayed arguments with my wife over and over in my mind. I worried about the mortgage and obsessed about my most complicated patients. I felt confused and tired. Why couldn't I just close my eyes and fall asleep? My brain was always in overdrive. I couldn't stop it.

At work, I was tired but functional. I began seeing more and more patients suffering from fibromyalgia. I remember looking at one particular patient's chart and reviewing the list of symptoms she had checked off:

Trouble sleeping: Yes
Joint pain: Yes
Abdominal pain and nausea: Yes
Itching: Yes
Depression: No
Joint swelling: No
Restless feelings in the legs: Yes

I walked into the room, and attempting to be reassuring, I introduced myself as Dr. Dryland, the new rheumatologist from Yale. She shot me a look that said she didn't care about my credentials—she cared about answers. Her history and exam were straightforward. I hated telling my new patient that she had fibromyalgia. I couldn't tell her why she had it, but I explained that her muscles likely hurt because she was either stressed or depressed. She just wanted to know how to find relief from the pain. I offered her what little I could, one prescription for pain medication and another to help with sleep. She shook her head and said she had already tried both of those prescriptions, and they didn't help. She questioned how stress could cause such severe pain. "I don't know," I said. "Nobody knows. I'm sorry. I wish I could help."

During the early years of my medical practice, I watched sick and desperate patients walk into my office, willing to do anything to get better. I remember how desperate I was for some sort of medical epiphany on those tired, pain-filled days and nerve-racking, sleepless nights as my own symptoms persisted. One day something clicked—an unnerving realization that my symptoms were almost identical to the ones I saw in my fibromyalgia patients. As I started asking my patients more questions about their sleep—the racing mind, the itching, the hot and cold sensations, the intense restless feelings in their legs, and even the violent jerking at night—I quickly understood that I was on the same path—the same slippery slope to full-blown fibromyalgia that these patients had traveled. I knew there must be something that triggered these common symptoms in their bodies and in my own.

None of the rheumatologists I worked with had any real answers, and I began to interview all the doctors I knew about their views on fibromyalgia. Some of the physicians I talked to jokingly told me that fibromyalgia (fortunately) wasn't their problem. "*That* is the rheumatologist's problem to deal with," they would say. Some doctors even insisted fibromyalgia didn't really exist. They insisted that *those patients* weren't actually in real pain, they were just depressed. Other medical doctors confessed their belief that fibromyalgia shouldn't be treated outside the psychiatrist's office. Frustrated with their responses, I began investigating stress and how it might affect fibromyalgia.

I went back to my dermatologist to ask whether my itching could be related to stress instead of a rash. Finally, she took me quite seriously. She had seen patients scratch themselves raw when stressed. Yet not a single colleague or any doctor I interviewed could give me a plausible reason for the symptoms of fibromyalgia. I searched through my medical books, but all I found were recommendations on various medications to help with pain and sleep. Having already prescribed most of those, I knew that at best, they offered fleeting relief for only some people. After reviewing what little knowledge I had about fibromyalgia, I started to dig for more information.

The Search for Answers

I spent my life training to think like a doctor. I learned to rely on hard facts when making decisions. It's easy to understand that when a blood vessel to the heart gets blocked, a patient will have reduced blood flow to that area and have a heart attack. When a patient herniates a disc in her back, the subsequent pressure on a nerve will cause great pain. Modern medicine understands problems like these and as a result has developed effective treatments. But what about treating a problem for which there doesn't seem to be a readily understandable cause? Unfortunately, the prevailing response in healthcare regarding problems that can't be understood or explained is to disregard their existence.

In medical school, I was taught that when people are stressed or depressed, they can spend all day focusing on their bodies until they start to believe that they have painful problem areas. The take-home message from medical school was that fibromyalgia wasn't a real medical problem and therefore belonged in the realm of psychology. I was told to reassure these patients that everything would be fine if they would just get some psychological help.

As I struggled with my own fibromyalgia symptoms and those of my patients in the late 1990s, I started to understand why physicians avoided fibromyalgia patients whenever they could. There just wasn't a clear way to help these people. Fibromyalgia patients made physicians feel frustrated and inadequate.

Now I was the one suffering unexplainable symptoms. As a patient, I knew my symptoms were real. As a doctor, I couldn't explain them, and neither could anyone else. I felt completely alone. I had real symptoms and no science to explain them. I was at a personal crossroads in my career and my life.

My search for answers started close to home. I began asking more questions of my fibromyalgia patients. I asked about their marriages, sleep, jobs, kids, car accidents, restless legs, itching, foggy thinking, recent moves, finances, family history, child-hood experiences, and even their own beliefs about fibromyalgia. Their answers surprised me. It seemed like every major life change caused fibromyalgia. Many patients were just fine until their divorce, and then their symptoms began. For others it was a motor vehicle accident or work injury that seemed to trigger their symptoms. One patient insisted her rheumatoid arthritis, a painful swelling of the joints, had initiated her fibromyalgia. (This didn't make sense at the time because even after I treated her disease and the swollen joints subsided, her fibromyalgia symptoms persisted.) I discovered a similar pattern in other patients. Taking careful case histories, I could usually help my patients identify an initial traumatic event, injury, or sequence of events that likely initiated fibromyalgia. However, in most of these cases, the patient had already recovered from the initial event or injury. The painful divorce was years ago, the initial injury had healed, or the son was out of jail and doing better. What baffled me was that the fibromyalgia symptoms and pain continued and even grew worse long after the initial fibromyalgia trigger was gone.

In my own research, I found confirmation that increased levels of stress, traumatic injuries, and poor sleep were starting to be associated with the onset of fibromyalgia. Conversely, lowering stress levels and getting better sleep were known to help alleviate fibromyalgia symptoms. Throughout my review of the existing medical research on fibromyalgia, I found many reports of potential causes but little that explained the science behind the symptoms. I knew there had to be a central cause that could explain this otherwise baffling assortment of symptoms.

Adrenaline and the Autonomic Nervous System

I was intrigued by a 1998 study that identified abnormalities in the autonomic nervous system (ANS) of fibromyalgia patients. The ANS is a nerve and chemical circuit board connected to every part of the body. Think of it as an *automatic* nervous system. It automatically makes adjustments to heart rate, blood pressure, digestion, respiration, and other body functions in response to changes in the body's internal environment. The ANS consists of the sympathetic nervous system and the parasympathetic nervous system, each of which acts in opposition to the other. The sympathetic nervous system is closely correlated with the fight-or-flight response. When the brain senses any type of threat (psychological or physical), the sympathetic nervous system goes into action and floods the body with stress hormones that prepare it to respond to an emergency. The most commonly known chemical involved in this process is adrenaline (also known as epinephrine). We all know what it feels like to get an adrenaline rush—everything seems to speed up, and that's exactly what happens. Our heart rate and blood pressure increase to supply extra blood and oxygen to our muscles. Our pupils dilate for better vision. Our mind sharpens and focuses on the potential threat. Adrenaline is only one of many chemicals designed to help us respond to an emergency. Noradrenaline and dopamine are also released, stimulating a cascade of changes and chemical releases throughout the body. These chemicals are also referred to as catecholamines, neurotransmitters, and neurohormones. The changes initiated by these chemicals give us the strength and endurance to fight or flee in times of acute danger. Once the threat has passed, the parasympathetic nervous system helps return the system to normal by slowing the heart, lowering blood pressure, constricting pupils, and redirecting blood flow to our extremities. This balancing act between the sympathetic and parasympathetic systems is an integral part of the ANS.

In the 1998 study, Dr. Manuel Martinez-Lavin of the National Institute of Cardiology in Mexico City studied the ANS in thirty people with fibromyalgia and thirty people without fibromyalgia by monitoring heart rate variability. Typically, ANS activity fluctuates throughout the day for all sorts of reasons. Most of us can identify with rapidly escalating adrenaline levels in times of extreme stress but are generally unaware of the more subtle fluctuations caused by everyday stressors. Mild adrenaline releases take place when we stub our toe or run into an old friend at the grocery store. In contrast, the parasympathetic system takes over after a meal, making us tired so that the body can focus on digestion. In a twenty-four-hour cycle, ANS activity rises during the day and falls back down at night. This cycle of change is part of our natural circadian rhythm, allowing us to maintain a regular sleep cycle. In general, a person's sympathetic nervous system is more active during waking hours, and the parasympathetic nervous system takes over at night. This rhythm ensures that we are more alert during the day because of the elevated levels of adrenaline and other chemicals. As we begin to retire for the evening, these chemicals dissipate, reaching their lowest levels when we are in the deepest sleep.

In his heart rate variability studies, Dr. Martinez-Lavin discovered that people with fibromyalgia had higher levels of sympathetic nervous system activity overall. In other words, these patients had consistently elevated levels of adrenaline, as if their fight-or-flight response was always on high alert. He also found that the ANSs of the fibromyalgia subjects did not have the usual twenty-four-hour circadian rhythm. Their ANS activity remained elevated, falling only slightly at night as compared to the controls (figure 1). Dr. Martinez-Lavin suspected that this unusual cycle was directly associated with the sleep disruptions previously reported in fibromyalgia patients.

The Martinez-Lavin study uncovered an important common denominator. Most of my patients had experienced physical pain or a psychological stress prior to the development of fibromyalgia. What did car accidents, illness, sleep problems, and divorce have in common? Each of these situations causes stress, whether it is emotional stress, physical stress, or sleep-deprivation stress. Likewise, in each of these situations, the brain sends a warning to the ANS, activating the fight-or-flight response. Typically, once a threat has passed, the body's on-guard mode relaxes. However, it appeared that in fibromyalgia patients, the normal

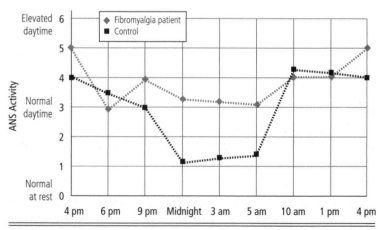

FIGURE 1 Elevated ANS Activity in Fibromyalgia Patients

balance between the sympathetic nervous system and the parasympathetic nervous system was chronically disrupted.

The Martinez-Lavin findings were confirmed in 2000 by the cardiologist Dr. Satish Raj and his colleagues at Queen's University in Ontario, Canada. Dr. Raj used a tilt table to study the ANS response of seventeen fibromyalgia patients and fourteen controls. In this test, patients lie on a table and are slowly tilted upward. A patient's physiological reaction to this stimulation provides important information regarding activity levels in the ANS. Dr. Raj confirmed that patients with fibromyalgia have a more active sympathetic nervous system—or fight-or-flight response. Dr. Raj wondered if this increased activity was the cause of fibromyalgia or simply the result of having fibromyalgia. Although I still wasn't sure how these studies explained the pain and other symptoms experienced by fibromyalgia patients, they certainly seemed to identify a significant imbalance in the body's normal functioning. Was this the systemic cause I had been looking for?

The Dopamine Connection

Another important piece of the puzzle fell into place when I met Dr. Andrew Holman, a rheumatologist at the University of Washington. We were among only a few clinical rheumatologists studying fibromyalgia. He was interested in the correlation between fibromyalgia and restless legs syndrome (RLS), another condition treated by rheumatologists. People with RLS experience an extremely unpleasant and difficult-to-describe feeling in the legs. Described by some as creeping, crawling, or itching, these sensations cause people to continually move their legs in an effort to avoid them. A disproportionate number of people with fibromyalgia also suffer from RLS. Dr. Holman recognized the overlap between RLS and fibromyalgia and wondered if fibromyalgia patients might benefit from the same drugs that help RLS patients. RLS, like fibromyalgia, also appeared to be associated with abnormalities in the ANS and elevated adrenaline levels. The most effective medications for RLS are drugs that mimic dopamine in the brain. Keep in mind that dopamine, like adrenaline, is one of the key chemicals the ANS uses to regulate body functions.

Dr. Holman's instincts helped turn the tide in the fight against fibromyalgia. In 2000, Dr. Holman published the first-ever study detailing how he successfully treated fibromyalgia patients with high doses of Mirapex (pramipexole), the same drug that alleviated symptoms of RLS. He later followed this initial study with a successful placebo-controlled clinical trial in 2005. After meeting Dr. Holman in 2001, I began prescribing these medications to my own patients. The results for those able to take this drug were phenomenal. One of my early patients shuffled in on a cane, hardly able to walk because of her pain. I started her on Mirapex, and within weeks, she literally threw away her cane!

I initially prescribed Mirapex to eighty-five patients with fibromyalgia and carefully tracked the results. Of this initial group, sixty-two were able to take Mirapex—albeit not always at the optimal dose due to some unpleasant side effects. In fact, the average dose people in that initial group were able to handle was less than half the optimal dose. Of the sixty-two who were able to take the medication, fifty-eight improved. Each one of these showed at least a 50 percent reduction in his or her pain score over the period covered by the study. Of the twenty-three patients who were unable to tolerate the medication, nausea was the chief problem reported. A few patients stopped taking the medication due to anxiety, poor sleep, confusion, or bad dreams. Most of the people who stopped taking the medication did so within the first week.

My patients who could tolerate Mirapex found that many or all of their fibromyalgia symptoms disappeared. For many of them, this was the first specific treatment that ever helped them. This was extremely exciting, but I also knew that Mirapex was not necessarily the cure for fibromyalgia. The high doses required for successful treatment can result in some intense side effects. Almost 30 percent of the people who tried Mirapex could not continue to take it for long enough to see results. That left too many of my patients out in the cold in terms of effective treatments. I also knew that I didn't want my patients to be dependent on a drug for the rest of their lives.

The successful treatment of fibromyalgia with a drug designed to simulate dopamine production in the brain confirmed my suspicions that an imbalance in the ANS—specifically an over-active fight-or-flight response—was somehow the root cause of fibromyalgia. If fibromyalgia could be virtually cured with a drug that mimics dopamine, then altered dopamine levels must play a central role in causing fibromyalgia! This latest revelation raised as many questions as it answered. What was going on here? Why did increasing dopamine, a chemical that should already be elevated due to a hyperactive fight-or-flight response, help alleviate a condition potentially caused by the fight-or-flight response? It was a seemingly unrelated study that helped me answer these questions.

In the late 1990s, Dr. Nadège Altier and Dr. Jane Stewart of the Center for Studies in Behavioral Neurobiology at Concordia University in Canada were studying the role of dopamine as an analgesic (pain reliever) in the body's pain-suppression system. As a chemical messenger, dopamine has many important functions in the body. A lack of dopamine in one part of the brain leads to the movement problems and tremors seen in Parkinson's disease. Increased levels in another part of the brain lead to feelings of pleasure associated with the brain's reward pathways. A specific type of dopamine naturally filters (and thus blocks) pain signals that would otherwise reach the brain. The role of dopamine in blocking painful sensations is so powerful that most prescribed narcotics inhibit pain, in part, by increasing dopamine activity in the brain. Dr. Altier and Dr. Stewart were specifically studying the role of dopamine in the ANS's fight-or-flight response by reviewing existing research and conducting their own studies.

Have you ever gotten an injury that didn't actually hurt until several hours later? Most of us have heard stories of people who experience traumatic injuries but claim that they didn't feel any pain until later. It turns out that dopamine provides significant pain relief at the time of the injury. When someone is injured, the fight-or-flight response kicks in, elevating dopamine levels to help ensure that excessive pain doesn't get in the way of the person's ability to either fight or flee. In 1999, Dr. Altier and Dr. Stewart studied the association between acute stress and pain suppression by enlisting some unsuspecting laboratory rats. Lowered into water, the rats were forced to swim for their lives, with no opportunity for escape. The researchers removed the frightened rats after a period of time and measured their pain response by injecting a needle into a tender paw. The rats didn't flinch. The forced swimming fully engaged the rat's fight-or-flight response, causing the ANS to release dopamine, adrenaline, and other neurohormones designed to protect the rats in times of danger. While adrenaline helped the rats swim harder and faster, elevated dopamine protected them from immediate pain in the same way that someone in a bad car accident doesn't always feel a broken bone right away.

Dr. Altier and Dr. Stewart continued to investigate the degree to which dopamine levels were related to diminished pain responses in the laboratory rats. In a subsequent test, they artificially elevated the rats' dopamine levels by giving them a drug instead of forcing them to swim. Once again, the scientists found that increased dopamine levels provided the same pain relief as the natural stress-induced dopamine. They also studied what happened if the stressed rats were deprived of dopamine (by giving them dopamine-blocking drugs) and then subjected to painful stimuli. They found that when the rats were deprived of dopamine, the usual stress-induced pain-blocking mechanism seen in previous tests did not exist. This particular test confirmed that dopamine was the key chemical responsible for blocking pain in times of acute stress. This finding also helped explain why high doses of Mirapex alleviated or eliminated symptoms of fibromyalgia in my patients.

Subsequent studies in 2000 and 2001 further revealed the link between dopamine depletion and fibromyalgia. Researchers at the Universidade Federal do Rio Grande do Sul in Brazil and at the University of Zulia in Venezuela took the initial rat studies a step further. Whereas Dr. Altier and Dr. Stewart studied rats exposed to acute stress, these next two studies measured the impact of chronic stress and the subsequent pain response in rats. It turns out that when rats are exposed to chronic stress, they start to lose the pain protection previously provided by dopamine. If the rats are exposed to stress on a daily basis for an extended period of time, they develop hypersensitivity to pain in much the same way that people with fibromyalgia have an increased awareness of pain. Pain medications also proved less effective than normal in chronically stressed rats. Similar findings were reported from studies run at a variety of other labs. Many of these studies paid special attention to those areas of the rat brain where dopamine activity regularly intensifies in times of acute stress. In stressful situations, dopamine levels increased and clearly afforded the rat protection from pain. However, under chronic stress, dopamine levels greatly decreased—not just to normal levels, but to less-than-normal levels. With depleted levels of dopamine, the rats lost their natural ability to filter pain signals and were more sensitive to mild pain stimuli than would normally be expected. Interestingly, these studies indicated that while dopamine becomes ineffective, adrenaline remains a powerful component of the stress response. Although the rats were lacking in dopamine, they continued to exhibit the signs of stress prompted by elevated adrenaline levels.

A Complete Picture

Science had not let me down. The rat studies were the final piece of the puzzle. Earlier studies provided proof that an overactive fight-or-flight response was closely linked to fibromyalgia. The rat studies demonstrated exactly how this connection worked. Designed to protect us from pain in the short term, an extended activation of the fight-or-flight response constantly depletes our supply of dopamine. Our body normally replenishes dopamine while we sleep. The Martinez-Lavin study provided evidence that fibromyalgia patients often have a disrupted sleep cycle. Without restorative sleep, dopamine production doesn't keep up with the increased demands of an overactive fight-or-flight response. A decreased supply of dopamine creates hypersensitivity to pain and other sensations.

The rat studies also answered another important question: Why do people with fibromyalgia continue to experience symptoms once the initial stress is gone? The stressed-out rats used in those studies continued to show a heightened response to painful stimuli for as long as four weeks after the stress was alleviated. This explained why fibromyalgia might persist long after patients have resolved the initial event or events that triggered fibromyalgia in the first place. Although the initial stressor is gone, the pain from fibromyalgia continues to keep the fight-or-flight response on high alert, further disrupting natural sleep patterns. This chronic activation of the fight-or-flight response continues to burn through any dopamine produced by the body. Once this happens, fibromyalgia becomes self-perpetuating, creating a vicious cycle that is hard to escape.

Final confirmation of the link between dopamine and fibromyalgia came in 2006 when Dr. Patrick Wood of Louisiana State University announced the results of his research on dopamine depletion in the brains of fibromyalgia patients. One of the world's leading dopamine researchers, Dr. Wood designed a system using PET scans to study dopamine levels in the brains of fibromyalgia patients. The PET scans allowed Dr. Wood to accurately measure dopamine metabolite levels in the brain. He was able to conclusively demonstrate that dopamine metabolite levels are consistently lower in patients with fibromyalgia when compared to people without fibromyalgia. Dr. Wood also demonstrated a reduced capacity for dopamine synthesis in the very areas of the brain that require dopamine in order to properly process pain signals.

Let's take a closer look at how altered levels of dopamine affect people at different stages of stress.

Figure 2 presents three scenarios. In the first, dopamine serves as a filter, selectively blocking out miscellaneous sensations so you can concentrate and get things done. Under normal circumstances, you never feel any sensations to the fullest extent. All day long, you are filtering out the touch of your glasses and your socks and the hum of your refrigerator. If you stub your toe, it definitely hurts, but not nearly as much as it

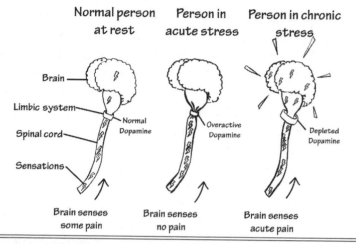

FIGURE 2 The Effects of Dopamine Depletion

would without the filtering action of dopamine. The second illustration demonstrates what happens when you experience acute stress, such as in the event of a serious car accident. The brain responds to the situation by increasing dopamine and blocking incoming sensations so that pain won't get in the way of a fight or an escape. In the third scenario, the brain has been under stress for so long that dopamine has become depleted, and the brain is suddenly bombarded by hundreds of unwanted and even painful messages. Although people often focus on the pain associated with fibromyalgia, all of your sensations become amplified once your dopamine levels run low. You lose the ability to selectively filter things out, and the world you live in dramatically changes.

I quickly realized that in order to help my patients, I would have to draw from many different disciplines. For centuries, science-driven Western medicine and spiritually based Eastern healing therapies have existed in opposition to one another. Western medicine focused on the tangible body, whereas Eastern medicine focused on the intangible mind. Western medicine has given us flu shots, chemotherapy, polio vaccines, and Tylenol. Eastern medicine has given us meditation, yoga, tai chi, energy healing, and acupuncture. By its very nature, fibromyalgia shatters the barrier between these distinct bodies of knowledge. If there was ever an illness that proves the power of the mind-body link, it is fibromyalgia.

What I saw next was that fibromyalgia can be reversed. The balance of the ANS can be restored, and people can once again lead healthy, active lives. Once I made use of my newfound knowledge with my patients, most of them felt better within weeks. In addition to working on reversing the causes of each person's fibromyalgia, I continued to prescribe medications that would help with pain, depression, and fatigue. Many patients just needed to give themselves time to heal and find out what was activating their fight-or-flight response. Most of the time, just understanding their situation helped patients feel better. Over time, my own symptoms disappeared, and I became more determined than ever to help people with even the most severe cases of fibromyalgia. I have learned that just as every patient has a different story of how he or she developed fibromyalgia, each one has a different path to recovery. Despite these differences, there is a consistency in fibromyalgia's root cause and a predictable set of steps that lead to recovery.

Remember Sophie, the patient I described at the beginning of this book? Sophie was lucky that she came to see me at the beginning of 2005. Several years earlier, I would have told her exactly what she didn't want to hear. I would have looked at her chart, reviewed her tests, and sadly told her that she had fibromyalgia. I would have explained that fibromyalgia is a syndrome, which means that it is a set of commonly associated symptoms rather than a specific illness. I would have told her that the medical community doesn't really understand what triggers fibromyalgia, what causes the pain, or why it doesn't go away. The best I could have offered would have been a vague hope that maybe someday we would know more about fibromyalgia.

Fortunately for Sophie, she came to see me after I had already helped a lot of other people recover from fibromyalgia. After reviewing her medical background and current symptoms, I did diagnose Sophie with fibromyalgia. I didn't, however, give her the grim prognosis that I described above. Instead, I carefully explained what causes fibromyalgia, where the pain comes from, and more important, I explained how she could move beyond fibromyalgia.

Her mouth dropped open, and she stared at me. "Are you telling me that I have fibromyalgia but that I can *get better*?" she asked in disbelief.

"Absolutely," I said.

"Do you mean that I can feel good enough to have children someday?" she asked, tears welling up in her eyes.

When I said yes, she wanted to know what was going on with the rest of the world.

"How come I haven't read a single thing that said I could get better? How come nobody has explained it like *this*?"

If you can relate to Sophie's pain, you should find inspiration in the second part of her story. I first met Sophie in February. She started to feel better almost as soon as she began following the program we developed together. Each day, a piece of her life fell back into place. First, her fatigue went away. She felt as if an enormous fog had lifted from her entire body. She still had pain, but daily activity was a little easier. Life now felt a little bit lighter. Gradually, she regained her independence and could drive her car, shop for groceries, and prepare a meal to share with her husband. Sophie found joy in everything that had once seemed mundane. By May, she had her first pain-free days in over a year.

She continued to work hard and make slow but steady progress. It wasn't always easy, and she had to make some tough decisions along the way. Slowly, she let thoughts about a bright future seep back into her mind. She started making plans without worrying about whether she would feel good enough to follow through on them. By October, Sophie knew she had made it. She had taken her life back, and never felt so good to simply be alive.

In a Nutshell . . .

- Fibromyalgia isn't forever—you can recover!
- People with fibromyalgia have an overactive sympathetic nervous system, also known as the body's fight-or-flight response. An overactive fight-or-flight response results in the continual release of adrenaline, dopamine, and other important stress-related hormones. If this elevated fight-or-flight activity continues, dopamine will become depleted.
- Disruptions in your sleep cycle (which you may or may not be aware of) prevent dopamine from being replenished at night.
- When your body experiences fight-or-flight fatigue, dopamine loses its effectiveness as a filter. It's like taking out earplugs at a rock concert and discovering that the music is so loud, it hurts. Once you lose the protection of dopamine, a pain blocker, all of your sensations (pain or otherwise) are suddenly amplified.
- The pain caused by depleted dopamine continues to trigger the fight-or-flight response, and fibromyalgia becomes a self-perpetuating illness.
- There is a solution to fibromyalgia. With knowledge and an effective treatment plan, you can rebalance your nervous system and reverse the fibromyalgia cycle.

CHAPTER 3

Understanding the Cause

Imagine that it is late at night and your car has broken down on a dark and unfamiliar side street. You get out of the car and start walking toward a gas station you passed a few blocks back. You hear footsteps rapidly approaching from behind and instinctively quicken your pace. Your heart beats faster as your mind starts analyzing the possibilities. Who's behind me? Are they going to hurt me? If they get too close, should I run?

Even before you start consciously processing the situation, your brain senses a potential threat and automatically activates the fight-or-flight response. A rush of adrenaline results in an almost instantaneous rise in blood pressure, heart rate, respiration, and blood flow to the muscles. All of your senses are heightened. You listen closely. If you need to run or even fight, your body is ready. Less obvious than the adrenaline rush, dopamine levels also rise. In the event of an injury, elevated levels of dopamine will prevent pain from getting in the way of a fight or an escape. If there is really a threat to your life, this unconscious activation of the fight-or-flight response might be the one thing that helps you survive.

In the last chapter, I described how chronically stressed lab rats developed a hypersensitivity to pain that could last up to four weeks after the stress was alleviated. These rats essentially developed fibromyalgia because their fight-or-flight response was repeatedly activated on a daily basis. Even though there are many different fibromyalgia triggers, the underlying cause is the same for everyone. Whether it is a divorce or a car accident that starts it all, the physiological cause responsible for fibromyalgia is a depletion of dopamine in the central nervous system. While circumstances that lead to dopamine depletion vary widely, they also fit into a specific and predictable road map. In this chapter, I'll explain in more detail how fibromyalgia is initiated, what triggers it, and what doesn't. I'll also explain why some people get fibromyalgia while others with similar circumstances seem to be immune. By the end of this chapter, you will have a good idea of what initially triggered your fibromyalgia. You will also have a solid understanding of the secondary factors that are keeping you trapped in the fibromyalgia cycle.

Fibromyalgia and the Fight-or-Flight Response

In order to better understand fibromyalgia in humans, let's take a closer look at how the fight-or-flight response operates. The fight-or-flight response is the most important survival instinct we have. Each and every experience we have is evaluated by our brain as a potential security threat. When the brain senses a threat, the fight-or-flight response goes into action. So why has this system gone awry for so many people? Why has our most important survival tool become responsible for so much pain and misery? The fact is that although our brain is extremely adaptive and capable of tremendous cognitive feats, it was wired for survival in a more primitive world.

How often do you look at the complicated lives that kids lead today and think about how much simpler life was when you were growing up? Isn't it amazing how quickly the pace of life can change in a single generation? In contrast, the fundamental biological mechanism of the fight-or-flight response has not changed for thousands of generations. The human fight-or-flight response evolved for use in life-threatening situations, such as an unexpected showdown with a saber-toothed tiger or possibly a late-night encounter with a threatening stranger. The fight-or-flight response was designed for infrequent use, making it safe for the body to rely on a potent mix of stress-related hormones to put our systems on high alert. Once the threat passes, the physiological reactions associated with the fight-or-flight response should subside, allowing the body to return to equilibrium.

As humans continued to evolve, we developed a more sophisticated brain capable of conscious thought and language. This clearly had its advantages. Thanks to human ingenuity, most of us have enough food to eat and a warm place to sleep. What more could a species want? The gift of language that defines us as an evolved species came with a serious downside, too. While language gives us the ability to think, analyze, speculate, and compare, it also allows us to worry, stress, fret, and obsess. Language facilitated logic, and as we all know, logic can be used constructively or destructively. Instead of living in the present moment, we can now thoroughly analyze the past and consciously worry about the future. Once humans developed the capacity for abstract thought, an entirely new set of fight-or-flight triggers came into being.

The human brain cannot tell the difference between a physical threat and a psychological threat; either is capable of activating the fight-or-flight response. Take a moment to imagine the last time you had an argument with someone you cared about. Remember what you said to one another and how it made you feel. As your mind replays this argument, can you start to feel your adrenaline rising? If the argument left you with enough of an emotional memory, you might even start to feel your heart rate and breathing quicken. This is the way that everyday events, some of which take place only in your thoughts, tip the balance of the autonomic nervous system toward fight-or-flight mode.

The Slippery Slope to Fibromyalgia

The human nervous system is not one that fares well when suffering from fight-or-flight response fatigue. The tremendous thinking capacity of the human mind combined with today's fast-paced, technology-driven, overloaded society has enormous implications. Think about how many so-called emergencies and seemingly potential disasters come up on a daily basis. Our action-packed lives come at a cost. We simply don't take the time to slow down anymore. Rather than taking an after-lunch siesta, we rush to the next task. Instead of being used only in true emergencies, the fight-or-flight response continually engages as we multitask our way through each day. Sometimes, we even consciously summon the extra burst of adrenaline needed to make it through the afternoon with a strong cup of coffee. Even when we are driving from one place to the next, we are busy analyzing, thinking, and processing all the thoughts and reactions that have bombarded our system that day. Many of those thoughts have the potential to keep our fight-or-flight response on a hair trigger. Perhaps all it takes is someone cutting us off in traffic to catapult our bodies into a full-blown fight-or-flight response. And then what? We can't fight it, we can't run—we're stuck stewing in our own brew of hormonal juices.

The body is remarkably resilient. It can continue functioning for a long time in less than ideal circumstances. There are signs of wear and tear—we feel tired, we catch colds more easily—but we keep going because the demands of modern life don't let up. It's no surprise that the stress of today's fast-paced world is implicated in the leading causes of death and illness—heart attacks, stroke, and even cancer. We're all aware of these risks, but we generally operate under the assumption that they won't happen to us. In addition to these commonly known risks, people who live life in a state of high alert for long enough may find themselves on the slippery slope to fibromyalgia. A lot of people might have even had a glimpse of fibromyalgia and not recognized it. Consider the following scenario:

John is the director of advertising at a busy public relations firm. He works long hours and has a stressful commute at the beginning and end of each day. Fortunately, John makes enough money that his wife doesn't work, and at the end of each day, he comes home to a nice dinner with his family. One afternoon, John's sister calls to tell him that their father is in the hospital after being involved in a bad car accident. The following weeks are more stressful than usual, and John has trouble sleeping. During the day, his attention is still fully focused on work, and it is not until he lies down at night that he has time to really think about his father. Instead of falling asleep, his mind starts to race as he analyzes the possible outcomes. After a few weeks of bad sleep, John starts waking up each morning feeling more stiff and tired than usual. A long-forgotten sports injury suddenly starts aching again, and the muscles in his shoulders and neck feel exceptionally tight and sore. His fight-or-flight response is now on a hair trigger. He is easily irritated by his children, expresses annoyance at the slightest provocation, and argues with his wife over nothing in particular. Fortunately for John, his father improves, life returns to normal, and those additional aches and pains quickly fade from his mind. He did, however, dip his toe ever so slightly into the murky abyss of fibromyalgia.

As we learned in the rat studies, too much stress over an extended period of time can reduce dopamine levels in the brain, resulting in hypersensitivity to pain. John experienced this on a mild level, as people do from time to time. Many of us live our adrenaline-filled lives on a slippery slope that can lead to fibromyalgia. So what makes the difference? Why do some people develop fibromyalgia while others seem to tackle the stress of daily life or even traumatic events with resilience? Much like any illness, it's hard to say why some people are susceptible while others remain resilient. However, as with any other illness, a combination of genetic tendencies, personal experiences, and even personality types play a role.

I once knew a woman who was going through a difficult separation from her partner. Her reaction to the stress was to sleep as much as possible. Sleep, if it is truly restorative, allows the body to rebalance, refresh, and restore important supplies of dopamine. Compare this woman with someone who finds it impossible to sleep given the same set of circumstances, and it's easy to see why one of them would be more likely to develop fibromyalgia. In John's case, what if he had learned his wife was having an affair shortly after his father's accident? Would that have pushed him over the edge? Or what if he already suffered from a painful illness himself? Maybe his father's accident would have been the last straw. The stories of what leads to fibromyalgia are as unique as the people who tell them. The one thing that's true in virtually all of these accounts is that once the fibromyalgia cycle gets initiated, things can go downhill rapidly.

The Fibromyalgia Cycle

As we discussed earlier, when I was first trying to understand fibromyalgia, I was extremely confused by the fact that a lot of my patients with fibromyalgia had already recovered from the event, injury, or illness that first triggered the syndrome. Why didn't the fibromyalgia go away once the initial stress dissipated? I eventually realized that people with persistent fibromyalgia are stuck in a vicious cycle. If the elevated fight-or-flight activity associated with the onset of fibromyalgia continues for long enough, depleted levels of dopamine are less and less effective at blocking pain and other uncomfortable sensations. The pain, confusion, and fatigue of fibromyalgia trigger additional stress and worse sleep—all of which keep the sympathetic nervous system in a continual state of arousal. The spiral can continue indefinitely, leading in many cases to devastating consequences and severe fibromyalgia.

Take, for example, the case of a young woman who gives birth to her first child. After a few weeks of euphoria, poor sleep and stress begin to take their toll. An already troubled marriage is strained by the demands of a new baby, and the young mother finds herself in the throes of postpartum depression. She and her husband have recently moved to a new city, and she doesn't have any friends or family to ease the transition to motherhood. The crying baby, the stressful marriage, and feelings of despair and loneliness initiate the fibromyalgia cycle. Her body, already strained by a difficult pregnancy, begins to ache more and more each day as her dopamine stores are depleted. She is exhausted but finds it difficult to sleep even when the baby is resting. She enters the fibromyalgia cycle, and without any change in her circumstances, her symptoms quickly spiral out of control (figure 3).

You can generally isolate the trigger responsible for your case of fibromyalgia by looking back at the events that took place in your life anywhere from a few months to two or three years prior to noticing your symptoms. At times, it can be hard to even figure out what that triggering event must have been. After all, the potential sources of stress, pain, and sleep disruption are innumerable. The experience you identify as your triggering event may have been the last in an already long list of potential triggers. You may end up concluding that the injuries from your car accident ultimately pushed you over the edge. Would that event have affected you in the same way if you were not already dealing with an emotionally painful divorce? Although it is impossible to predict what combination of circumstances or experiences will trigger fibromyalgia for any particular

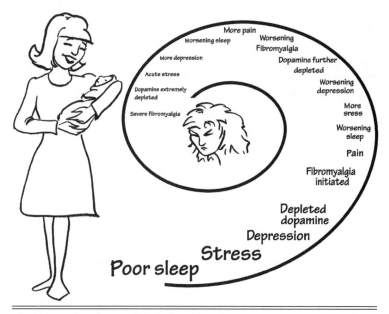

FIGURE 3 The Fibromyalgia Cycle Initiated

individual, the triggers themselves are predictable and easy to categorize. The three categories of triggers for fibromyalgia are

- sleep disruption
- physical pain
- psychological stress

Most people with fibromyalgia will experience triggers from more than one of these categories. Physical pain and psychological stress initiate the fibromyalgia cycle by keeping the body in a constant state of high alert. Remember, the human brain does not distinguish between the stress generated by physical or emotional pain. It will interpret either one as a threat and automatically trigger the fight-or-flight response. Disrupted sleep, in combination with these other triggers, can seal your fate by depriving your body of the opportunity to restore the supply of dopamine and other important chemical substances. In order to recover, you must first recognize any potential triggers. Be sure to read through the entire list of fibromyalgia triggers. My patients sometimes mistakenly dismiss a potential trigger before they have taken the time to truly consider whether it might be applicable.

There are primary and secondary triggers. A primary trigger will initiate fibromyalgia. Secondary triggers continue the cycle even after the primary cause fades away. Although it is important to understand the initial event that started the fibromyalgia cycle, the key to finding relief is understanding what keeps you trapped in the cycle (figure 4).

Sleep Disruption

In the 1970s, scientists discovered that they could create the symptoms of fibromyalgia in healthy volunteers simply by

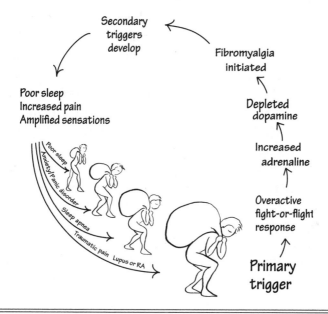

FIGURE 4 The Fibromyalgia Cycle Deepens

disrupting the deepest stages of sleep. After a few nights of interrupted sleep, volunteers complained of aching muscles and overwhelming tiredness. Another study analyzed the sleep patterns of fifty women with fibromyalgia. This study discovered that whenever any of these women suffered a poor night of sleep, it was almost invariably followed by a day of intensified pain. Does this sound familiar?

Poor Sleep

Over 90 percent of fibromyalgia patients also suffer from a sleep disorder. Many of the sleep disorders result directly from an overactive fight-or-flight response. When the fight-or-flight response is engaged, sleeping becomes much more difficult. This makes a lot of sense, because the fight-or-flight response was designed to protect you from life-threatening situations. It certainly wouldn't be safe to fall asleep if your life were truly at stake. Instead, your mind takes advantage of the lack of distractions to analyze problems and develop new strategies for success. As you fall asleep at night, does your body suddenly jerk back awake? These little jolts of adrenaline are the body's way of saying, "Wake up! It's not safe to sleep right now."

Some fibromyalgia patients find it difficult to sleep when they are in pain, because they find it hard to relax enough for sleep to take over. Other fibromyalgia patients are able to fall asleep easily enough, but their sleep patterns are disrupted, preventing them from getting good-quality sleep. Regardless of why fibromyalgia patients don't sleep, the end result is the same. A lack of deep, restorative sleep deprives the body of an opportunity to replenish an overused supply of dopamine.

Sleep Apnea

Unlike insomnia or other sleep problems, sleep apnea can be the sole cause of fibromyalgia. With sleep apnea, a breathing obstruction or even a complete cessation of breathing occurs during sleep. Deprived of oxygen, the body automatically stops sleeping in order to begin breathing again and then returns to a lighter stage of sleep. Sleep apnea not only prevents you from achieving quality sleep, it's also a powerful trigger of the fight-or-flight response. There's nothing like nearly suffocating every night to drive your adrenaline levels right off the chart. And that's exactly how your body reacts whenever your oxygen level plunges because you've stopped breathing. Your body literally snaps out of any stage of sleep in order to start breathing again. This can happen hundreds of times each night!

I believe that sleep apnea is an important (and often hidden) cause of fibromyalgia in men. Altogether, I have found that approximately 5 percent of my fibromyalgia patients have been laboring for years with undiagnosed sleep apnea. That percentage is much higher for men, as well as for anyone who's overweight. It seems that in men, sleep apnea is one of the most important triggers for fibromyalgia. My suspicions about the relationship between sleep apnea and fibromyalgia in men were confirmed by a study conducted at the Fitzsimons Army Medical Center Rheumatology Clinic. Researchers examined all new fibromyalgia patients for sleep apnea. After testing, 2.2 percent of the female patients were diagnosed with sleep apnea, which is similar to the prevalence rate of 1.2 percent in the general population. In contrast, an incredible 44 percent of the male subjects in the study suffered from sleep apnea, as compared with 3.9 percent in the general population. This is similar to the percentage I have seen in my own practice.

Most people with sleep apnea don't realize they have it until they're diagnosed. What they do know, however, is that they regularly wake up very tired, possibly with a headache, and that they sometimes even awaken in pain or in a state of confusion. These people also have a tendency to gain weight and suffer from high blood pressure, and they often contend with a host of other serious health problems. If you suspect sleep apnea might be involved, ask your healthcare provider about being tested for this important hidden cause of fibromyalgia.

Restless Legs Syndrome

Over 30 percent of people with fibromyalgia also suffer from restless legs syndrome (RLS), an unpleasant sensation in the legs alleviated only by movement. The uncomfortable and uncontrollable jerking leg and arm motion associated with RLS is directly related to an overactive sympathetic nervous system. At first, RLS may appear to be more a symptom than a cause of fibromyalgia. In most cases, that's probably true. However, once people with RLS acquire one or more of the other triggers described here, RLS can start to act as a contributing trigger in its own right. RLS symptoms are often worse at night, and the associated sleeplessness will certainly exacerbate fibromyalgia. Also, in those cases in which a diagnosis of fibromyalgia is not entirely certain, the presence of restless legs tends to alleviate any doubts.

Physical Pain

Any type of chronic pain can trigger fibromyalgia. Apart from suffocating nightly as a consequence of sleep apnea, there's nothing better at getting the attention of your fight-or-flight response than pain. People who start off with a painful condition, such as lupus, rheumatoid arthritis, or chronic back pain, are all the more likely to develop full-blown fibromyalgia in a relatively short period of time. These people already have pain, so any depletion of dopamine will make their pain worse, and their symptoms will quickly become unbearable. Other painful conditions, such as tendonitis or bursitis, are not necessarily severe enough to initiate fibromyalgia. However, these can quickly become secondary triggers that contribute to the fibromyalgia cycle as soon as fibromyalgia is initiated. An uncomfortable case of tendonitis will morph into an extremely painful and disabling condition once the body's pain signals become amplified. Listed below are some specific physical conditions that have a proven track record of causing fibromyalgia.

Chronic Painful Disorders

People with painful conditions such as osteoarthritis, lupus, rheumatoid arthritis, and chronic low back pain are at risk of developing fibromyalgia because their bodies are already subjected to constant physiological stress. For reasons that probably are starting to sound familiar to you, people who suffer with painful arthritis in their joints are halfway to getting fibromyalgia as well. In fact, studies have shown that 20 percent of people with nearly any type of rheumatic disease meet the diagnostic criteria for fibromyalgia. With their already elevated adrenaline levels (raised in response to the arthritic pain), these people also have a fight-or-flight response that's on a hair trigger. A bout of depression or a poor night's sleep might be all it takes to kick the adrenaline system into chronic overdrive. What this amounts to, unfortunately, is that the margin of safety for patients who already suffer with painful conditions is slim. Any further dopamine depletion will likely result in fibromyalgia.

Painful Trauma

Any painful trauma can increase the chance of developing fibromyalgia. I've treated many patients who were able to handle poor sleep or stressful situations just fine until they suffered some sort of physical trauma. Car accidents resulting in whiplash or other painful conditions are commonly reported as an initial fibromyalgia trigger. This is probably because car accidents are one of the most common causes of traumatic injury. Anything that causes pain can trigger the fight-or-flight response for an extended period of time. The potential for developing fibromyalgia is compounded if more pain, poor sleep, depression, and/or stress follow. A painful trauma is all the more likely to cause fibromyalgia if you already have problems with stress, depression, or sleep.

Hypermobility Syndrome (Double Jointedness)

People with lax or loose joints often complain of pain similar to the pain caused by fibromyalgia. These pains may simply stem from the trauma their loose joints regularly experience.

A 2005 study conducted by researchers at Marmara University in Istanbul, Turkey, evaluated 151 women with and without fibromyalgia for signs of hypermobility. Sixty-four percent of the women with fibromyalgia had hypermobile joints, as compared with 22 percent of women without fibromyalgia. In my own practice, I've found hypermobile joints to be a major contributing trigger of fibromyalgia. People who are double jointed are likely to get fibromyalgia if they also have any of the other causes noted in this section.

Psychological Stress

It probably comes as no surprise that chronic stress is one of the most common triggers of fibromyalgia. In fact, in combination with poor sleep, it rates as one of the leading triggers. If your life seems overwhelming and chronic stress is inescapable, an elevated fight-or-flight response is inescapable. Stress also causes blood pressure and pulse rate to rise, contributing to hypertension, high blood pressure, and other serious medical conditions. Stress is often associated with heart disease, ulcers, and deficiencies in the immune system. It is also closely linked to almost all the causes listed in this chapter. Pain certainly causes stress, as does illness, grief, or a hectic schedule. Aside from elevated levels of daily stress, the following psychological conditions are closely associated with fibromyalgia.

Anxiety and Panic Disorders

Individuals suffering from a combination of chronic anxiety and panic disorders generally face more serious consequences than do those who simply deal with high levels of stress. In my own practice, I have documented a strong link between anxiety, panic disorders, and fibromyalgia. How can you tell the difference between the two? Typically, panic attacks involve the sudden onset of intense fear or terror. Generalized anxiety disorder, on the other hand, is more constant, characterized by chronically high levels of worry and anxiety that are difficult to control and typically result in significant distress and impairment.

In addition to the obvious psychological strain, people who suffer from these mental disorders also tend to manifest physical symptoms. Many patients suffering from panic disorders experience intense chest pain despite having no obvious heart problems. What's most likely happening is that the panic disorder has left the patient effectively stuck in the fight-or-flight response. The associated depletion of dopamine intensifies awareness of pain in the area of the chest where connective tissues come together. In fact, fibromyalgia is sometimes first detected in patients seeking medical attention for a sudden intensification of their chronic chest pain.

Unfortunately, after some of these patients are told there's actually nothing wrong with their hearts, they may start to think they're crazy and overreacting. The pain they're experiencing is 100 percent genuine. These patients feel the connective tissue in their chest more than others do because they're stuck in fight-or-flight mode and have a depleted dopamine supply. During the panic attack, they further exhaust their dopamine supply and subsequently feel as if they are having a heart attack.

Depression

Although depression more often manifests as a symptom of fibromyalgia, it certainly has its place as a fibromyalgia trigger. Depression is a general term that can include intense depression, a more temporary response to grief, chronic depressed mood, and what has been termed "normal" depression. Depression is entirely normal and is woven into the fabric of each person's lifelong development, surfacing periodically in response to all manner of life events. Think back to a time when you were depressed, and you can probably recall how you experienced excessive worry or anxiety during that time, along with altered moods, sleep difficulties, and/or fatigue.

I believe that when we're depressed, the brain acts on the assumption that something is wrong and responds by activating the fight-or-flight response. If you're chronically depressed, your fight-or-flight response is already overactive. Anything else that causes your adrenaline to improperly cycle will have an exaggerated effect and could easily trigger fibromyalgia. Contrary to popular opinion, you do not have to be depressed to develop fibromyalgia. It is not uncommon for people with fibromyalgia to subsequently experience depression, as fibromyalgia can be such a life-altering illness. Although the exact brain chemistry has yet to be determined, altered or depleted dopamine is certainly believed to play an important role in depression. The depleted dopamine associated with fibromyalgia may leave you more susceptible to depression. Once you develop depression, it becomes a secondary trigger of fibromyalgia.

Posttraumatic Stress Disorder

Posttraumatic stress disorder (PTSD) refers to any stress that remains long after the trauma that caused it has receded into history. PTSD is a very common trigger of fibromyalgia—so much so that for years, many in the medical community operated under the assumption that all patients with fibromyalgia had been abused or had experienced extreme trauma at some point. This is simply not true. Many PTSD patients have had prolonged traumatic experiences in which they have felt trapped for months or years. PTSD can also result from a bad childhood, abusive relationship, or a prolonged stressful situation in the face of some other difficult living circumstance. Whenever we experience anything of the sort for an extended period of time, our bodies become accustomed to operating in habitual fight-or-flight mode.

Patients with PTSD often describe getting intense adrenaline rushes whenever they're having a flashback. It is a tragedy that people who have experienced a severe trauma are faced with reliving it over and over again. The body actually experiences the trauma anew, using up dopamine with each succeeding flashback. These flashbacks can be triggered at any time by thoughts, discussions, random events that strike some familiar chord, or even just the mere anticipation of the anniversary of the event in question.

I've tended to many patients who've insisted they've managed to put their PTSD and the associated flashback episodes behind them through years of therapy. Unfortunately, even after escaping such terrible circumstances, the fight-or-flight response often remains on a hair trigger, affecting the perception and experience of all future situations.

Bipolar Disorder (Manic Depression)

Bipolar disorder is a serious mental illness in which manic episodes are interspersed within a more general condition of depression. Although not commonly thought of in these terms, patients with bipolar disorder live with an extremely overactive fight-or-flight response. There are many people with bipolar disorder who have enjoyed tremendous success, including world leaders, respected thinkers, and famous artists. Their increased adrenaline levels likely provide the driving force behind their accomplishments. But for all their successes, many of these people probably kick their legs at night, sleep poorly, and ache all the time.

With bipolar disorder, manic episodes are characterized by exceptionally elevated or irritable moods accompanied by unusually high self-esteem, a reduced need for sleep, bursts of chattiness, racing thoughts, and/or unrestrained involvement in pleasurable activities, resulting in long-term consequences. In these people, adrenaline levels are always elevated. In my opinion, bipolar disorder is one of the hardest fibromyalgia triggers to resolve. However, it can be successfully treated with a combination of medication and psychotherapy.

Why Are Women More Susceptible Than Men?

The triggers described above are universal. So why are women nine times more likely to develop fibromyalgia than men? No one's really sure why women are more susceptible to fibromyalgia, but I suspect it has something to do with the different ways men and women deal with stress. Men and women both have a fight-or-flight response, but researchers at the University of California, Los Angeles's Department of Psychology have proposed that women have different tendencies with regard to the fight-or-flight response. They have suggested that women are less prone to fighting or fleeing and more inclined to "tending." From an evolutionary standpoint, if women always chose to fight or flee, they would risk leaving their offspring vulnerable to attack. In order to safeguard their offspring, women may have a genetic tendency to stay in place and attempt to resolve difficult or emotionally painful situations. This caregiving instinct led Dr. Shelley Taylor of the UCLA Department of Psychology to describe a woman's fight-or-flight response as the "tend and befriend" response.

In light of this theory, consider how men and women might respond differently to the same upsetting situation. If men are angry or upset, they may stomp out of a room, go for a run, engage in contact sports, or pick a fight in a bar. Although some women may show these responses as well, others are more inclined to stay in the unpleasant situation, trying to sort it out. Rather than acting on their emotions, as their male counterparts often do, they may internalize their feelings and dwell on upsetting situations for longer periods of time. The ensuing internal monologue may repeatedly trigger the fight-or-flight response. Women, therefore, may be more vulnerable to fibromyalgia due to their genetic tendencies as caregivers.

Another part of the answer may lie in the results of a London study from the 1970s in which three physicians at the National Hospital for Nervous Diseases developed a computer-assisted technique for monitoring people's breathing without disturbing them. Part of their study involved documenting the differences between male and female sleep patterns. Their research proved that it is much easier to interrupt a woman's sleep than a man's. This is likely a very important component of a woman's genetic makeup, allowing her to respond quickly to her child's cry at night. This genetic difference may be one more reason that women are more susceptible to fibromyalgia. If women are naturally lighter sleepers, they may be more predisposed to sleeping poorly during times of stress, one of the key triggers of fibromyalgia.

In a Nutshell . . .

- The fight-or-flight response is our most important survival instinct. However, it evolved for infrequent use—such as a showdown with a saber-toothed tiger—making it safe for our bodies to rely on a potent mix of stress-related hormones in emergency situations.

- Once humans developed the capacity for language and abstract thought, an entirely new set of fight-or-flight triggers came into being. The human brain cannot tell the difference between a physical threat and a psychological one. Either one is capable of activating the fight-or-flight response.

- In today's stressful world, most of us suffer from some degree of fight-or-flight fatigue. It's hard to say why some people are susceptible to fibromyalgia while others remain resilient. As with any other illness, a combination of genetic tendencies, personal experiences, and even personality types play a role.

- Sleep deprivation, psychological stress, and physical pain are the three categories of fibromyalgia triggers. Psychological stress and physical pain trigger an overactive fight-or-flight response. A lack of deep, restorative sleep deprives the body of the opportunity to replenish its supply of dopamine.

- Fibromyalgia triggers may be primary or secondary in nature. Secondary triggers continue the cycle even after the primary trigger disappears.

- Once fibromyalgia is initiated, a vicious cycle ensues. The pain, confusion, and fatigue of fibromyalgia trigger additional stress and poor sleep—all of which keep the sympathetic nervous system in a continual state of arousal. The spiral can continue indefinitely, leading to devastating consequences and severe fibromyalgia.

- Women are more susceptible to fibromyalgia than men due to genetic differences in both their fight-or-flight response and their tendency to be easily aroused from sleep.

CHAPTER 4

Fibromyalgia and Other Conditions

On Cindy's first visit to my office, she could barely walk. Hunched over from pain, she leaned heavily on a cane for support as she shuffled from the waiting room into the examining room. Her daughter stood nearby, having driven her mother to my office and filled out the paperwork on her behalf. Cindy could not drive or hold a pen long enough to fill out the patient questionnaire. There wasn't much of Cindy's body that didn't hurt. Getting out of bed and making it to my office were Herculean efforts for her. Cindy felt like she was ninety years old, but in reality she was a forty-seven-year-old single mom with severe fibromyalgia.

Cindy had suffered from fibromyalgia for almost a decade before I met her. Her symptoms started in 1996, after she suffered a mild stroke. Exhausted and achy, she felt like she had a bad flu that never went away. Her memory was awful, and she had trouble concentrating for any length of time. Like many other fibromyalgia patients, it took years for Cindy to get an accurate diagnosis, as doctors confused her symptoms with other conditions. Cindy was initially diagnosed with hypothyroidism, a disease with symptoms similar to those of fibromyalgia. Her doctor prescribed a medicine to supplement the suspected deficiency in thyroid hormone. When her symptoms failed to improve, her doctor responded by prescribing a higher dose. Her doctor continued to increase her dose until Cindy landed in the emergency room with a wildly erratic heartbeat. Another doctor subsequently diagnosed her with chronic fatigue syndrome. A third doctor told her she suffered from clinical depression and wanted to prescribe antidepressants. The problem was that Cindy didn't feel depressed. She hurt everywhere and was really, really tired, but she didn't think she was depressed. As her pain and fatigue increased, Cindy's workweek decreased from forty hours to thirty hours, and finally down to no more than twenty hours in good weeks.

Eventually, a rheumatologist diagnosed Cindy with fibromyalgia. Although this doctor finally got the diagnosis right, his prognosis was dead wrong. After telling Cindy that she had fibromyalgia, he told her there was nothing he could do for her symptoms except prescribe some pain medication. She was totally dispirited. A formerly active woman, Cindy remembers packing up all her hiking guides and giving away her camping equipment. She looked in the mirror and no longer recognized the tired and crippled woman who inhabited her formerly healthy body. After meeting Cindy, I confirmed her diagnosis, but I explained that she could definitely recover from fibromyalgia. We developed a recovery plan for her, and within a very short period of time, Cindy threw her cane away and never looked back. Today, Cindy is as happy and healthy as she's ever been.

Cindy's story is far from unusual. Doctors and patients often confuse the symptoms of fibromyalgia with many other conditions. In turn, there are several conditions commonly mistaken for fibromyalgia. Fibromyalgia patients have always had to serve as their own best advocates. This isn't likely to change in the near future. In most cases, it will be up to you to determine which of your symptoms are from fibromyalgia and which indicate that another condition should be tested for. In order to do this, you'll need to learn more about how fibromyalgia affects your body. You already understand that fibromyalgia results from a problem in the autonomic nervous system (ANS). This chapter more fully explains how the body interprets sensory signals once you have fibromyalgia. It also describes the way fibromyalgia complicates other diagnoses and provides information on medical conditions commonly linked to or confused with fibromyalgia. By the end of this chapter, you should more fully understand which of your symptoms stem from fibromyalgia and which ones might be attributable to another medical condition. If you have fibromyalgia or think you do, it is critically important to consider whether other conditions may be responsible for some of your misery. Resolving any underlying medical conditions will be an integral part of your recovery.

The Pain Threshold

As we've discussed, fibromyalgia patients have depleted dopamine levels, so dopamine cannot filter and block pain sensations as it normally would. The point at which something hurts is the moment the sensation exceeds the pain threshold. The amount of dopamine in a person's brain determines his or her pain threshold. Let's assume that dopamine normally blocks half of all the sensations we experience. If a painful injury registers 10 on the severity scale, a healthy person with a normal level of dopamine feels a pain severity of 5 (figure 5).

A moderate fibromyalgia sufferer with a reduced pain threshold feels an unbearable pain severity of 8, and a severe fibromyalgia sufferer with virtually no pain threshold remaining feels a suicidal pain severity of 10. When pain reaches a severity of 8 or 10 in fibromyalgia patients, visits to the local emergency room (ER) are not uncommon.

These desperate trips to the ER rarely lead to relief. Instead, these experiences often deepen the frustration and confusion the person already feels. Typically, the ER doctor on duty will be unable to provide either an explanation or proper treatment, and neither will the surgeon. Following a few tests, the patient may be told that there is nothing structurally wrong, since all test results look perfectly normal. Although that may be true, it doesn't help the person with fibromyalgia feel any better. Neither will the token prescription for pain relievers written by the bewildered physician. In some cases, the patient in the ER

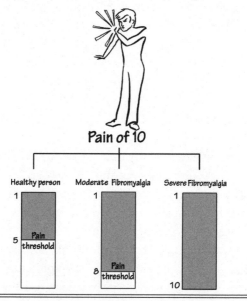

FIGURE 5 Ouch! That Hurts!

may never have heard of fibromyalgia before, and he or she will leave the ER in pain and with no rational explanation. The pain the patient experiences, however, remains 100 percent genuine.

I often tell my patients and their spouses to imagine that they've just worked all day cleaning out the garage. Both are sure to have minor muscle aches and strains by the end of the day. But the person with normal dopamine levels will feel these minor problems only slightly—and only when he or she happens to move in a certain way over the next couple of days. The fibromyalgia sufferer, on the other hand, may end up incapacitated—restricted to a recliner and covered with ice packs for the next week or so. Both likely have a similar assortment of strained muscles—the only difference being that the person with fibromyalgia has to deal with a greatly amplified pain signal (figure 6).

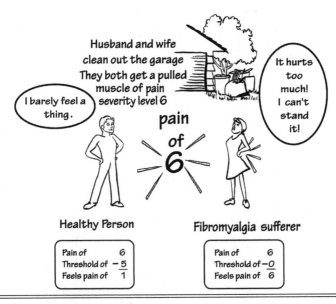

FIGURE 6 It Hurts Too Much!

Does Fibromyalgia Harm My Body?

Most of my patients feel that fibromyalgia must cause harm to their bodies. That's easy to understand, because that's how it feels. It can seem like your body is falling apart. Fortunately, in spite of the pain and misery inflicted by fibromyalgia, this disruption in your ANS doesn't directly harm your body. Although your body hurts like hell, fibromyalgia does not cause long-term, irreversible damage to your body. It's important to believe that once you follow the steps to recovery, you will have a healthy body waiting for you.

There are, however, some indirect consequences of suffering from fibromyalgia for an extended period of time. Although fibromyalgia doesn't directly harm your body, the associated pain and fatigue can stop you in your tracks. As your activity level decreases in response to pain and fatigue, your muscles will get tight and become more painful. Poorly toned muscles are also more susceptible to small tears and injuries that will feel anything but small to you. Think back to your activity level before you developed fibromyalgia. Everyone with fibromyalgia slows down, and there are unavoidable consequences associated with decreased activity levels. Fortunately, none of these consequences cause permanent harm to your body.

Fibromyalgia Exacerbates Other Conditions

Fibromyalgia doesn't actually cause other health problems; it just uncovers problems that have always existed and would have continued to go unnoticed had you not been afflicted with fibromyalgia. Fibromyalgia operates like a giant magnifying glass, making you aware of imperfections in your body that you might not have previously taken the time to notice. Virtually every other malady—be it an allergy, lower back pain, endometriosis, a rash, the flu, or carpal tunnel syndrome—suddenly jumps from the unconscious to the conscious. Anything and everything that's even slightly abnormal will be sensed earlier, felt more intensely, and linger longer. When you have fibromyalgia, it's more important than ever to recognize and treat other problems that are adding to your misery.

Two of the most common problems exacerbated by fibromyalgia are allergies and infections. Many fibromyalgia patients who have never so much as sneezed at a bit of dust or pollen before are shocked to discover they have allergies. For those who have a history of allergies, the symptoms become more intense and are often harder to treat. I see a greater proportion of patients using nasal inhalers, taking antihistamines, and getting allergy shots. Is fibromyalgia causing the allergies? Of course not, but once dopamine is depleted, even the slightest itching of the eyes or postnasal drip results in intense discomfort. The symptoms cause a much greater proportion of patients to seek medical care for their allergies.

The same is true of infections. Fibromyalgia does not cause infections. However, as is the case with any stress-related illness, your immune system will not operate at peak efficiency, so infections will more easily occur. What's more, you're certain to feel every infection much more intensely when your dopamine is depleted. Fevers and chills will feel more intense, muscle aches from the flu may become disabling, and the urge to cough will increase as secretions in the throat are felt more intensely. Even though fibromyalgia can't be blamed for *causing* your infection, it does make a substantial difference all the same—namely, you'll feel the infection sooner, the symptoms will be more intense, the infection may seem to run a longer course, and it will be harder to resolve all the symptoms.

Not only does fibromyalgia exaggerate symptoms, it also complicates the treatment of just about any ailment.

This pattern repeats itself over and over again in fibromyalgia. As the fibromyalgia cycle continues its downward spiral, it seems like more and more things are going wrong with your body. Medication lists grow longer as additional health problems surface. These could include a heightened awareness of not only allergies and infections but also many other conditions, including the following:

- chronic sinus pain
- yeast infections
- painful fluid retention in the ankles and feet (edema)
- headaches (including migraines)
- plantar fasciitis (tendonitis in the arches of your feet)
- many other instances of tendonitis or bursitis
- growing pains
- hypoglycemia
- endometriosis
- painful menses
- fibrocystic breast disease
- frequent colds
- morning stiffness
- sunburns
- muscle twitching
- insect bites
- ingrown toenails
- adverse reactions to medications
- dry skin
- sore throat
- premenstrual syndrome
- temporomandibular joint syndrome
- dry eyes and/or mouth

Mind you, none of these things in their own right are pleasant. With fibromyalgia, they can become downright unbearable.

These are real medical problems, and you should actively work to resolve them, but never forget that every real problem is greatly amplified by fibromyalgia. Consider how fibromyalgia can complicate the treatment of people who suffer from carpal tunnel syndrome. Carpal tunnel syndrome is a common, painful condition caused by compression of the median nerve in the wrist. Symptoms start gradually and include pain, weakness, or numbness in the hand and wrist. As pressure on the nerve increases, symptoms may also include tingling and decreased grip strength. Mild cases of carpal tunnel syndrome are easily treated through rest, ice, and anti-inflammatory medications. More severe cases may require surgery. If the patient has fibromyalgia (diagnosed or not), it can be all but impossible to tell how much of the pain is directly attributable to carpal tunnel complications and how much is simply due to a decreased pain threshold caused by fibromyalgia.

Let's assume that three people have identical cases of mild carpal tunnel syndrome (figure 7). Under normal circumstances, they would each have a pain severity of 3. If we assume that the normal pain threshold is 5, then a healthy person would not even notice a mild case of carpal tunnel syndrome. However, someone with mild fibromyalgia has a decreased pain threshold and feels mild pain. On visiting a doctor, that person would be instructed to use a brace when doing repetitive work or sleeping. Someone with severe fibromyalgia and a greatly lowered pain threshold feels severe pain. It's likely that the person could have surgery for the exact same problem that would cause no pain in a person with normal levels of dopamine. Will the surgery be successful?

A successful surgery doesn't always completely solve a problem, but it relieves it to the point where subsequent pain

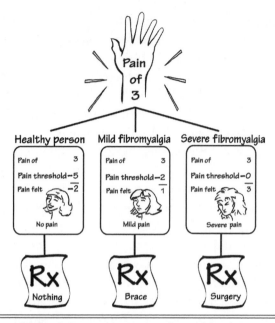

FIGURE 7 Fibromyalgia Exaggerates Carpal Tunnel Syndrome

signals are below the pain threshold. However, with lower levels of dopamine, any residual nerve compression following surgery can still cause pain because the hypothetical patient with fibromyalgia doesn't simply have carpal tunnel syndrome. The correct diagnosis for this person's pain is carpal tunnel syndrome amplified by fibromyalgia. This is an important but often missed distinction.

Postoperative problems aren't specific to carpal tunnel syndrome. Many fibromyalgia patients report dissatisfaction following surgeries and other invasive procedures designed to help alleviate pain. Many problems require surgical correction. If you have a condition for which surgery is necessary and you suspect that this particular problem is one of your fibromyalgia triggers, then you should not delay. However, if the pain is mild and surgery is at all optional, I encourage you to focus instead on the program outlined in part 2 of this book. Once you are successful in raising your dopamine levels, you might find that you don't need surgery any longer.

Distinguishing Fibromyalgia from Other Problems

There are many illnesses that have similar symptoms and may in fact overlap with fibromyalgia. However, before I describe conditions commonly confused with fibromyalgia, I want you to understand how to distinguish fibromyalgia symptoms from other problems. It is extremely important to learn what problems are primarily caused by the fibromyalgia and what problems are separate and may require additional treatment.

The most important thing to understand about fibromyalgia symptoms is that they vary only with the fibromyalgia causes. Your fibromyalgia symptoms are directly linked to your fibro-myalgia triggers: poor sleep, psychological stress, and physical pain. Although you have chronically low dopamine levels, they are probably relatively stable most of the time. However, they will fluctuate easily in response to any of the triggers. If you experience more stress or your sleep problems get worse, dopamine levels will plummet, and your symptoms will get worse. Conversely, if you take a vacation, reducing your stress and increasing the quality of your sleep, you will feel better, as your dopamine levels will have a chance to replenish. Your fibromyalgia symptoms will *always* vary with your particular triggers. The symptoms from other conditions will also be felt more intensely as your fibromyalgia flares. However, the symptoms of these other medical conditions will always be present, even when you have a good day and your other fibromyalgia symptoms are mild.

As an example, many patients with fibromyalgia also have osteoarthritis, a condition resulting from wear and tear on joint cartilage. If you suffer with both conditions and your back starts hurting, how do you know whether it is the fibromyalgia or the osteoarthritis? First, review the triggers of each condition. Fibromyalgia symptom severity varies with stress and poor sleep, while osteoarthritis symptom severity varies with the weather and your activity level. Did you do too much, or did you have a poor night of sleep followed by a stressful day? If you are feeling well rested and refreshed but your back still hurts, then osteoarthritis is probably the culprit. It's not always easy to tell because sometimes it can be both. A flare-up of low back pain from cleaning out the garage can worsen sleep and certainly increase stress. In this case, your fibromyalgia and osteoarthritis may both be causing you substantial pain. But if you pay attention to your body, you will slowly learn to distinguish between fibromyalgia and other conditions.

In the end, you are the only one who really knows how your body feels. Due to the variety of symptoms that come and go on a daily or weekly basis, only you can know whether your symptoms are from fibromyalgia or from another medical condition. Sorting this out and gaining knowledge about what is actually happening in your body are critical parts of your recovery from fibromyalgia. You'll have an opportunity to list your symptoms and develop a detailed case history in chapter 5. For now, I want you to learn more about other conditions that might cause some of the same symptoms experienced with fibromyalgia.

Conditions Most Commonly Confused with Fibromyalgia

The three medical conditions most commonly confused with fibromyalgia are lupus, multiple sclerosis, and chronic fatigue syndrome. These three diseases have two things in common with fibromyalgia: they are all difficult to diagnose, and each one can prove very challenging to treat. The symptoms also mimic fibromyalgia and in some cases overlap it. To add to this confusion, these diseases cause chronic pain and discomfort and in some cases may actually be the initial fibromyalgia trigger. In this case, both conditions would then exist simultaneously.

Lupus

Lupus is a chronic autoimmune disease in which the immune system mistakenly attacks healthy cells and tissues in the body. Lupus is a genetic condition, and only people who inherit the genes for lupus are susceptible. Lupus is a serious illness that may include fever, rashes, painful joints, and damage to the major organs, including the kidneys, liver, heart, lungs, and brain. Unlike fibromyalgia, lupus causes inflammation that results in swollen joints. Lupus can also be subtle and cause only pain and fatigue. Just like fibromyalgia, symptoms can come and go, and new symptoms can appear at any time. There is no single test to diagnose lupus, and some people suffer for years without knowing what is wrong. Lupus is not reversible, but certain medications can decrease the abnormal immune response.

The painful symptoms and stress associated with lupus are powerful triggers for fibromyalgia, and many people suffer from both. Approximately 30 percent of lupus patients are also diagnosed with fibromyalgia, making it very confusing for any physician to sort out symptoms and provide relief. There are many more undiagnosed cases of lupus with subsequent fibromyalgia, because most physicians stop looking for another problem once they diagnose lupus. At least 75 percent of my lupus patients also suffer from fibromyalgia. I have found that much of the suffering typically associated with lupus actually stems directly from fibromyalgia. Lupus sufferers, for example, often have cognitive problems ranging from difficulties with concentration to simple forgetfulness to psychosis and hallucinations. If seizures, psychosis, or hallucinations are present, fibromyalgia is surely not to blame. But when it comes to the simple confusion that so many lupus sufferers report, the subsequent development of fibromyalgia is almost always to blame. The primary lupus symptoms are listed below. You'll notice many symptoms that don't actually overlap with fibromyalgia that can help distinguish the two conditions.

Primary Lupus Symptoms: painful, swollen joints; muscle pain; fever with no known cause; red rashes on the face and elsewhere; chest pain with deep inhalations; hair loss; pale or purple fingers or toes; sun sensitivity resulting in rashes; swollen glands; fatigue; mouth ulcers; and leg swelling.

Multiple Sclerosis

Multiple sclerosis (MS) is another confusing and difficult to diagnose illness. Although scientists are not totally sure what causes MS, most believe it is an autoimmune disorder that disrupts communication between the brain and other parts of the body. It can cause overwhelming fatigue, numbness, pain, visual abnormalities, and other neurological symptoms. The initial symptom of MS is often blurred or double vision, red-green color distortion, or even blindness in one eye. Most MS patients experience muscle weakness in their extremities and find coordination and balance difficult. These symptoms may be severe enough to make walking or even standing difficult. Approximately 50 percent of people with MS experience difficulties with concentration, attention, memory, and poor judgment.

MS commonly affects women in their twenties to forties and is often very difficult to diagnose. There isn't any one feature of MS that is unique to this disease, but vision or bladder abnormalities often suggest MS should be considered in the diagnosis. The symptoms of MS are erratic and can come and go in different combinations as the disease progresses. For many patients, heat exacerbates the symptoms. At times, MS seems to go into remission. MS is diagnosed by a neurologist through a combination of tests, including MRI scans and a sample of spinal fluid. Depending on the stage of the disease, the diagnosis can be an educated guess rather than an absolute certainty. As in lupus, specific medications are used to dampen the immune response. Although the stress and pain of MS could be a trigger of fibromyalgia, there does not seem to be a significant overlap between these two conditions. The primary symptoms of MS are listed below.

Primary MS Symptoms: muscle weakness; moderate to severe pain; inability to coordinate muscle movements; continually contracted muscles; tremors; speech disturbances; vision disturbances; dizziness; bladder dysfunction; bowel dysfunction; cognitive difficulties; and fatigue.

Chronic Fatigue Syndrome

Chronic fatigue syndrome (CFS) is characterized by profound, unrelenting fatigue and shares many symptoms with fibromyalgia. In addition to fatigue, CFS patients have short-term memory or concentration problems, muscle pain, multijoint pain without swelling or redness, headaches, and sleeping problems. No one knows for sure what causes CFS, but for years, experts have tried to link this condition to a lingering viral infection. Most CFS patients identify a viral infection or other illness as the definitive trigger of their condition. CFS remains a diagnosis of exclusion, as patients are only diagnosed with CFS if their symptoms are not attributable to any other medical cause or condition.

Many experts consider CFS and fibromyalgia to be the same diagnosis with different names. This simply isn't true. Although many symptoms overlap, there are also important differences between fibromyalgia and CFS. The symptoms of CFS also include sore throat, tender lymph nodes, and extreme exhaustion following exercise. CFS patients also experience frequent fevers and swollen glands. Although fibromyalgia patients may occasionally experience these symptoms as the result of overlapping conditions, a sore throat, tender lymph nodes, swollen glands, and fevers are not inherently characteristic of fibromyalgia.

The most important difference between fibromyalgia and CFS is that the fatigue from fibromyalgia varies with the fibromyalgia triggers, while the fatigue from CFS does not. In my own practice, I have occasionally found fibromyalgia patients who were misdiagnosed with CFS simply because they didn't exhibit the classic fibromyalgia tender points. There's also a good chance that the poor sleep and other problems associated with CFS serve as fibromyalgia triggers, leaving some people to suffer from both conditions. The most common symptoms of CFS are listed below.

Primary CFS Symptoms: fatigue for six months or longer with no known medical reason; short-term memory or concentration problems; sore throat; tender lymph nodes; muscle pain; multijoint pain without swelling; headaches of a new type, pattern, or severity; unrefreshing sleep; and postexertion exhaustion lasting more than twenty-four hours.

Other Conditions Confused with Fibromyalgia

Many other conditions are commonly confused with fibromyalgia. As I review these conditions, you will notice a consistent pattern. Not only does fibromyalgia mimic other diseases, but the suffering caused by many chronic diseases also triggers fibromyalgia. Many people can have both. Don't lose hope. Keep in mind that these diseases are often rare, while fibromyalgia is common. Many people who fear they have Lyme disease or rheumatoid arthritis will discover they have fibromyalgia instead. You can recover more easily from fibromyalgia than from many of these other conditions. This makes understanding the differences between fibromyalgia and other conditions that much more important.

Lyme Disease

Ticks carrying a specific bacterium transmit Lyme disease to humans through a bite. Ticks that transmit Lyme disease are found mainly along the East Coast and in midwestern states. The first sign of infection is usually a circular rash surrounding the bite. People with Lyme disease may also have signs of fatigue, chills, fever, headache, and muscle and joint aches. When caught in the early stages, the infection, which initially occurs at the site of the tick bite, is easily treated with antibiotics. If the infection, which does not always exhibit symptoms, goes untreated, it may spread to other parts of the body. These cases can be difficult to diagnose, as symptoms may be erratic and occur months or even years after the initial bite. Chronic Lyme disease can mimic fibromyalgia, presenting with fatigue, pain, and confusion. As the disease progresses, people may experience periodic episodes of arthritis, with severe joint pain and swelling. There can also be more serious problems, such as cardiac and neurological abnormalities. Specific lab tests and other findings are used by physicians to diagnose this infection. Almost everyone with Lyme disease recovers when treated with antibiotics. However, recovery may proceed slowly in cases that remain untreated for long periods of time. In some cases, Lyme disease may trigger fibromyalgia. This could explain the small percentage of people who are diagnosed with Lyme disease and are treated but continue to have ongoing, persistent symptoms.

Rheumatoid Arthritis

Rheumatoid arthritis (RA) is an autoimmune disease that causes painfully swollen joints and fatigue. People with RA may have fatigue, occasional fevers, and a general sense of not feeling well. RA can be treated most effectively when diagnosed early. Unfortunately, early RA is often difficult to diagnose. Symptoms vary from person to person and occur at different levels of severity. Some symptoms may not occur until the disease progresses. Symptoms can be confused with other types of arthritis and joint conditions, and it may take some time for other conditions to be ruled out. Although physicians can test for an antibody in the blood specific to RA, not everyone tests positive for this antibody. Left untreated, RA destroys the bone and cartilage in affected joints. Doctors treat RA with powerful medications to suppress the immune system in order to reduce painful inflammation and prevent joint damage.

If a doctor suspects that you might have fibromyalgia, you will be tested for RA in an attempt to rule out this painful disease. As a chronic and painful disease, RA can trigger fibromyalgia. However, there are several ways to distinguish the two conditions. Most notably, the joints affected by RA will appear warm and swollen, something that won't happen with fibromyalgia. RA also causes bumps around the joints called rheumatoid nodules. These bumps often occur just below the elbow joints. RA generally occurs in a symmetrical pattern, meaning that if one knee or hand is involved, the other one will be affected as well. The joints most commonly affected are the wrist joints and the finger joints closest to the hand.

Hypothyroidism

Hypothyroidism is a disease of the thyroid gland. Located at the base of your neck, the thyroid gland helps control your metabolism. With hypothyroidism, the thyroid gland stops making the correct amount of thyroid hormone, causing many body functions to slow down. People with a sluggish thyroid feel cold, tired, and constipated. They gain weight and move and speak slowly. They often have generalized muscular pain. Whenever someone experiences a combination of pain and fatigue not easily explainable by another condition, thyroid levels are checked through a common blood test. If your doctor suspects fibromyalgia, you should also be checked for hypothyroidism, which is easily treated by taking thyroid hormone medication. Discuss this possibility with your doctor if you feel very cold, experience rapid weight gain, or if your hair is brittle.

Neuropathy

Neuropathy means disease of the nerve. There are a multitude of problems that can affect nerve function, including infections, diabetes, autoimmune problems, vitamin deficiencies, and nerve compression. Some problems, such as peripheral neuropathy, are genetic in nature and can have severe body-wide consequences. Once a nerve is damaged, symptoms include pain, numbness, tingling, and even weakness. Neuropathy can be treated with medications, physical therapy, braces, or even surgery. Specific tests performed by a neurologist can help diagnose neuropathy and determine the appropriate course of action.

Some nerve problems are progressive in nature and start off with mild, undetectable damage to the nerves in question. People with mild abnormalities of their nerves may be years away from noticing their first symptoms. However, if you have fibromyalgia and your sensation threshold is lowered, you may quickly become aware of any mild nerve damage you might have. This explains the unusually high percentage of fibromyalgia patients who are also diagnosed with carpal tunnel syndrome or a mild generalized peripheral neuropathy (a disease usually affecting the nerves of sensation in the hands and feet). If you have neuropathy and fibromyalgia, each condition should be taken seriously. People sometimes assume that neuropathy is simply another symptom of fibromyalgia that they have to live with. This isn't true. Fibromyalgia does not cause neuropathy. Unfortunately, a formal diagnosis may be difficult to get for the relatively mild cases sometimes experienced by fibromyalgia patients. These cases may not feel mild to you, but that's often due to your heightened sensitivity associated with fibromyalgia. The typical tests used by neurologists may not actually detect neuropathy in its early stages. If you have symptoms of tingling or numbness in your hands or feet, talk to your doctor about the possibility of neuropathy. Even if your tests come back negative, you may still have mild neuropathy. In these situations, the symptoms will likely disappear as you start to recover from fibromyalgia.

Chronic Myofascial Pain Syndrome

Although fibromyalgia and chronic myofascial pain syndrome commonly overlap and are frequently confused with one another, they are distinct entities. Chronic myofascial pain syndrome results in localized pain rather than the diffuse pain that is common in fibromyalgia. People with this syndrome can generally identify specific areas of the body that are chronically painful. Myofascial pain syndrome is characterized by the development of taut bands of muscle, also known as trigger points. The pain from trigger points may be localized or refer to different areas in the body. Secondary complications can include increased pressure on nerves, muscles, bones, and organs. The painful areas associated with myofascial pain syndrome are often caused by injury, repetitive motions, lack of activity, tension, or poor posture and body mechanics. This condition differs from fibromyalgia in that the pain stems directly from problems in the muscles and connective tissues (fascia).

These two conditions not only frequently overlap but also may trigger one another. The painful symptoms of myofascial pain syndrome could certainly contribute to the initiation of fibromyalgia. On the other hand, the inactivity and poor body mechanics exhibited by fibromyalgia patients are both frequent triggers of myofascial pain syndrome. In fact, a high percentage of fibromyalgia patients have the trigger points associated with myofascial pain syndrome. There are some key features of each syndrome that make it easy to distinguish between the two. Fibromyalgia patients suffer from diffuse pain and chronic fatigue. Patients with myofascial pain syndrome have localized pain and do not suffer from fatigue. The morning stiffness and tender points common with fibromyalgia are not symptoms of myofascial pain syndrome. Furthermore, myofascial pain syndrome can be resolved through treating the source of the pain.

Appropriate treatments may include physical therapy, acupuncture, massage, chiropractic manipulation, or even surgery (if the condition warrants it). Since myofascial pain syndrome is treatable, it is important to distinguish between the diffuse pain characteristic of fibromyalgia and pain that results from an actual structural abnormality.

Dementia

As discussed earlier, fibromyalgia patients often experience some cognitive problems, commonly referred to as fibro fog. These frequent lapses in memory and inability to think clearly cause some people with advanced fibromyalgia to start wondering whether they might be suffering from dementia. Dementia is a brain disease affecting memory that is often associated with thinking and behavioral abnormalities. Most people think of Alzheimer's, a degeneration of the brain usually affecting the elderly, but there are many other causes of dementia. As people age, there is a normal slowing of cognitive and memory functions. Many of my patients with fibromyalgia feel that this is happening to them no matter what age they are. Most patients with fibromyalgia have problems with concentration and memory. Researchers who compared the cognitive problems of fibromyalgia patients with those of elderly people found that even though fibromyalgia patients exhibited problems with simple concentration and memory, they did not show the processing problems evident in some of the elderly patients. The reassuring news is that your concentration and memory problems are more directly related to your pain level than to any permanent pattern of cognitive impairment. Unlike the elderly, who often suffer from degeneration or disease in the brain, fibromyalgia patients have trouble with memory and concentration because their brains are stuck in an on-guard mode that is more concerned with survival than cognitive thinking. Even so, these particular symptoms can be very troubling for people who have to think on their feet, especially those with demanding cognitive and technical jobs.

Irritable Bowel Syndrome

Irritable bowel syndrome (IBS) is a common condition of the digestive system involving abdominal pain, heartburn, constipation, and diarrhea. The causes of IBS and fibromyalgia are remarkably similar. People who suffer from these conditions have nearly identical triggers, including stress, poor sleep, posttraumatic stress disorder (PSD), depression, and anxiety. In fact, a study found that 70 percent of fibromyalgia patients also have IBS, and 65 percent of IBS patients also have fibromyalgia. Despite this incredible overlap, these conditions are discrete entities. Your intestines have their own local nervous system that reacts in its own way to the increased adrenaline levels common to each of these conditions. IBS is essentially fibromyalgia of the bowel. However, the problems associated with IBS are caused by different chemicals than those implicated in fibromyalgia. Still, it's quite likely that the bowel, like the ANS, learns to behave in an abnormal and disconcerting manner from years of coping with an overactive fight-or-flight response. I mention this, as you will find your bowel symptoms also vary with your fibromyalgia triggers. I have found that some patients are more troubled by their IBS symptoms than their fibromyalgia symptoms. Treatments for IBS are designed to control the symptoms and usually involve dietary changes and medications for gas, constipation, heartburn, and other symptoms. Fortunately, many of the same steps you take to resolve fibromyalgia will help resolve your IBS problems as well.

Overlapping Imbalances

As you know, stress causes more problems than just fibromyalgia. The stressful triggers that lead to fibromyalgia will disrupt many other biochemical processes in your body. In particular, researchers have discovered altered levels of substance P, cortisol, and growth hormone, among others, in fibromyalgia patients. These imbalances have led to widespread speculation regarding the role of these substances in fibromyalgia. Although an imbalance in any one of these substances may contribute to your symptoms or cause other problems, none of them should be mistaken for causing fibromyalgia.

As researchers keep looking, they will find more and more imbalances in fibromyalgia patients. Each of these problems is indicative of a processing problem in the central nervous system. The research on fibromyalgia will continue to evolve, and new discoveries will cause people to speculate on the role each imbalance might play in causing fibromyalgia. Although this research is important, the speculation that it generates is currently getting in the way of treating fibromyalgia, as each of these substances plays only a small role in the big picture. Of all the imbalances involved, dopamine depletion is the key culprit when it comes to the cause of fibromyalgia symptoms. Furthermore, the true cause of fibromyalgia will never change. All these chemical abnormalities and varied symptoms are the end result of an overactive fight-or-flight response. Once you resolve the underlying cause of fibromyalgia, your system will once again find balance.

In a Nutshell . . .

- Fibromyalgia doesn't directly harm your body! Fibromyalgia lowers your sensation threshold and makes you hypersensitive to any problem—no matter how mild—that comes your way. Allergies, infections, headaches, and many other problems are made worse by fibromyalgia.

- Tight knots and stiff muscles may develop as your activity level decreases in response to increased pain and fatigue. Once again, these problems are greatly exacerbated by fibromyalgia.

- Fibromyalgia is commonly confused with difficult to diagnose illnesses that have similar symptoms. Doctors and patients most frequently confuse fibromyalgia with lupus, multiple sclerosis, and chronic fatigue syndrome.

- Some other overlapping and/or commonly mistaken conditions include Lyme disease, rheumatoid arthritis, hypothyroidism, neuropathy, chronic myofascial pain syndrome, and irritable bowel syndrome.

- A chronic and painful illness can actually trigger fibromyalgia, so some people suffer from fibromyalgia on top of another problem.

- Don't assume that every pain or symptom you have stems from fibromyalgia. Another condition may be responsible. Learn how to tell the difference between fibromyalgia symptoms and other problems. It is important to resolve any underlying problems that are adding to your misery.

- Fibromyalgia symptoms always vary with the fibromyalgia triggers. Increased stress or pain in combination with poor sleep causes fibromyalgia symptoms to flare. Decreased stress and improved sleep temporarily improve fibromyalgia symptoms.

- There are many systemic imbalances associated with fibromyalgia. In addition to dopamine depletion, altered levels of substance P, cortisol, and growth hormone have been found in fibromyalgia patients. All of these chemical abnormalities are the end result of an overactive fight-or-flight response. Once you resolve the underlying cause of fibromyalgia, your entire system will once again find balance.

CHAPTER 5

Do I Have Fibromyalgia?

I was tempted to start the book with this chapter because people are always anxious to find out if they have fibromyalgia. However, I've found that it takes a lot of background information before you can form an educated opinion about the root cause of your symptoms. At this point, you probably have a pretty good idea whether you have fibromyalgia. You may have already known that you had fibromyalgia, and now for the first time you understand how it actually works. Or perhaps you're surprised, because although you have all the symptoms and many of the triggers, no one has ever diagnosed you with fibromyalgia.

In the preceding chapters, you learned what fibromyalgia is, what causes it, how it can affect you, and how to identify other health conditions you might have. This chapter sets the stage for part 2 of this book, in which you will develop and implement your own recovery plan. First, I'll explain why the official diagnostic criteria for fibromyalgia make it so difficult to get an accurate diagnosis in anything resembling a reasonable amount of time. Then, I'll explain the diagnostic criteria that I use when examining potential fibromyalgia patients.

I'll help you develop your own case history so you can apply my diagnostic criteria to your situation. By the end of this chapter, you should have a good understanding of what initiated your case of fibromyalgia and what your current triggers are. Once you understand fibromyalgia in light of your specific triggers, you will be armed with the most powerful weapon I can give you: knowledge.

Outdated Diagnostic Criteria

Just about any physician who examines you for fibromyalgia is relying on outdated and misleading diagnostic criteria that largely miss the point. When the American College of Rheumatology (ACR) developed the diagnostic criteria for fibromyalgia in 1990, it didn't have a lot of material to work with. Although fibromyalgia was certainly becoming common, knowledge about the biological underpinnings of this illness was severely lacking. Diagnostic criteria are essentially a set of universal guidelines that physicians rely on to make objective and accurate diagnoses. But how do you develop diagnostic criteria for an illness you don't really understand? How do you give doctors a rule book for an illness that changes the rules with each patient? In 1990, the ACR did the best it could with the information at hand and developed a set of criteria that focused on what was apparently the defining characteristic of fibromyalgia: pain. Traditionally, physicians have used these criteria to make a fibromyalgia diagnosis. However, with the new information available on the causes and symptoms of fibromyalgia, these criteria are outdated and largely inaccurate.

According to the traditional criteria, a patient must first have a history of widespread pain. To be specific, the patient must have widespread musculoskeletal pain lasting longer than three months in all four quadrants of the body. In addition, the patient must experience pain along the axial skeleton (in the upper spine, breastbone, midspine, or low back). Think about this in light of what you now know about fibromyalgia. When a person first enters the fibromyalgia cycle, the amplified sensations may be moderate and will not necessarily spread throughout the body. In fact, pain might not even be one of the first symptoms of fibromyalgia for some people. It certainly wasn't in my case. However, according to the ACR criteria, the pain must be chronic before an illness can be considered fibromyalgia. The very nature of the official diagnostic criteria make it impossible to diagnose people at the very beginning of the fibromyalgia cycle. Once the pain can be described as chronic and widespread, fibromyalgia has gone on for way too long. Physicians need to start looking at the true causes of fibromyalgia in relation to amplified sensations rather than relying on chronic, widespread pain as their primary indicator.

The second diagnostic criteria regarding tender points is also problematic. According to this criteria, doctors must examine a patient for pain in eighteen different tender points across the body (figure 8). When a physician presses on each of these points with a specific amount of pressure, the patient must indicate that at least eleven of them are painful. These tender points are associated with areas where ligaments and tendons insert into bones. Everyone has some tenderness in these areas to start with. Many people with fibromyalgia experience an elevated awareness of tenderness or pain if a doctor starts poking and prodding these particular areas. However, there is no particular correlation between these specific points and fibromyalgia. People in the early stages of fibromyalgia may not experience any pain in the tender points on examination. As fibromyalgia progresses, pain signals are more easily

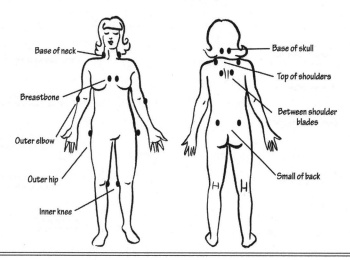

FIGURE 8 Possible Fibromyalgia Tender Points

triggered by even the lightest touch or slightest movement. Even then, the presence or absence of these tender points does not necessarily confirm or dismiss a fibromyalgia diagnosis. The symptoms of fibromyalgia vary on a daily basis, making it impossible to rely on criteria dependent on a single physical examination. Someone with fibromyalgia who had pain in seven of eighteen tender points on Tuesday may have pain in sixteen of eighteen tender points on Friday. His or her diagnosis would depend entirely on which day the doctor's examination took place.

If you dip a fishing net with large holes into the ocean, you're only going to catch fish that are too big to slip through the holes. The smaller fish will swim right through your net. This is essentially the problem with the current diagnostic criteria. The holes in the current diagnostic criteria are so big that an awful lot of fibromyalgia patients never get "caught." This explains why so many fibromyalgia patients suffer for years before receiving an accurate diagnosis. It is only after their fibromyalgia reaches the level of severity and intensity identified by the traditional criteria that they finally receive an appropriate diagnosis. As with any other illness, fibromyalgia patients recover much more easily when the problem is recognized early on, and the current diagnostic criteria prevent this.

I am certainly not the first to criticize the ACR criteria as a diagnostic tool for fibromyalgia. In 2002, an editorial in the *Journal of Arthritis and Rheumatism* noted that by focusing solely on pain, these criteria disregard many of the other symptoms associated with fibromyalgia, including fatigue, confusion, and sleep disturbance. I once treated a police officer who was unable to sleep because of the intense crawling sensations he felt all over his body. The sensations were greatly intensified whenever the officer was under stress, particularly if he'd recently had a lot of difficult interactions with the public or even with his sergeant. He also noticed that the crawling sensations decreased whenever he was away on vacation. He was beginning to think that perhaps he was allergic to his patrol car, his uniform, or perhaps even his house. He experienced these uncomfortable sensations primarily at night while he was home, and a naturopath diagnosed him as having multiple chemical sensitivity syndrome. He was encouraged to completely redesign his home to eliminate the offending substances. The officer had done it, and yet he was still miserable at night.

Understandably, he became more frustrated, and the problem only got worse as a consequence. He endured three more years of being tested by allergists, dermatologists, and neurologists, all to no avail. After all that, the officer's primary-care physician was at a total loss as to how to proceed. That's when he came to me, expecting yet another disappointment. I quickly saw that he suffered from stress, depression, and restless legs syndrome. What's more, he verified that his crawling sensations varied in step with these fibromyalgia triggers. As we know, in fibromyalgia the symptoms always vary with the triggers. When the triggers are reduced, the fight-or-flight response relaxes, dopamine is replenished, and symptoms diminish. That's why it came as no surprise to me that his symptoms improved whenever he was on vacation but worsened whenever stress increased.

I explained to him that fibromyalgia was the cause of his sensations and that this was a very curable situation. He was dubious at first—not surprising, given all that he'd already been through. I persuaded him to take a medication that would increase his dopamine levels. Even at a very low dosage, he was amazed to find that the crawling disappeared in just under a month. At this point, he understood that his problem related entirely to an imbalance in his autonomic nervous system (ANS), and he dropped the medication and started working on other techniques for minimizing stress and depression. Eventually, the crawling sensations disappeared. Although it was clear to me that the officer had fibromyalgia, he may never have been diagnosed according to the traditional criteria because he would not have exhibited the required tender points. It's likely that he would still be suffering from fibromyalgia if I hadn't seen the correlation between the fibromyalgia causes and his symptoms. It's possible that his fibromyalgia may have progressed to the point where he developed pain as well. If he was lucky, someone might have diagnosed him with fibromyalgia years later.

In order to diagnose my own patients, I have developed a new set of diagnostic criteria that accurately detect fibromyalgia in patients at any point in the cycle. Unfortunately, I am a rheumatologist, not a primary-care physician. I only see patients who have first been referred to me by their primary-care physician. This means most patients I see have had fibromyalgia for quite some time.

Creating a Case History

Given today's official diagnostic standards, you are in the best position to evaluate your symptoms as they relate to fibromyalgia. Your first task is to create your own fibromyalgia case history. You should follow the steps in this process even if you're already sure that you have fibromyalgia, and be sure to document your case history in writing. Creating a thorough case history will greatly help you develop and implement a recovery plan. Your case history will also be an extremely useful tool when working with healthcare providers in the future. Putting your case history on paper can provide physicians with some important insights about your particular case of fibromyalgia that might otherwise be overlooked.

Your case history should consist of a time line that traces your symptoms as they relate to life events, stress levels, sleep patterns, and medical history. This will help you identify the initial fibromyalgia triggers as well any additional triggers that are currently exacerbating your condition. Take a moment to review the primary fibromyalgia triggers. You'll want to keep these in mind as you develop your case history.

- Psychological Stress

    Elevated stress level
    Anxiety/panic disorder
    Depression
    Posttraumatic stress disorder

Bipolar disorder/manic depression
Other serious psychiatric disorders

- Physical Pain

  Chronic, painful disorder (common ones include lupus and osteoarthritis)
  Painful trauma (such as a car accident, injury, or even a repetitive motion problem)
  Hypermobility (double jointedness)

- Sleep Deprivation

  Insomnia
  Sleep apnea
  Restless legs syndrome

If you have only recently begun to suspect fibromyalgia, it shouldn't be too hard to develop a fairly detailed case history that documents changes in your health on a monthly basis. If you have had fibromyalgia for an extended period of time, creating a case history might seem daunting. Don't worry. Focus on three different time periods in your case history. The first of these is the beginning of the fibromyalgia cycle. Think back to your health state at the onset of your symptoms. Second, take note of any significant events, changes in health, improvements, or declines that have taken place in the intervening years. Finally, document the past twelve to eighteen months as thoroughly as possible. The past year of your life will provide the most important clues as to what is currently keeping you trapped in the fibromyalgia cycle.

The first question to ask yourself is "When did my symptoms start?" This seems like an obvious question, and you might think you know the answer. Regardless of what you already believe, take a moment to think carefully about the answer to this question. In the past, you might have assumed the fibromyalgia started when the pain started. Now that you understand fibromyalgia in a different light, think carefully about what symptoms might have preceded the pain. Perhaps there were some earlier indicators that your body was developing the hypersensitivity characteristic of fibromyalgia. Were your allergies worse that year? Did you have irritable, tender skin? Did you have unexplained aches or pains that seemed to come and go? If you have trouble remembering exactly what was happening in your life, talk to a friend or family member who might be able to help you remember. Friends and family members often can provide you with important insights into aspects of your life you might otherwise not have.

Once you think you know when your symptoms started, think carefully about what was taking place in your life in the preceding six months. Did you have an injury? a bout with depression? Were you sick? Was there a death in the family? Were you sleeping well? Did you have a baby, transfer to a new job, separate from your partner, or experience any other challenging emotional situations? Remember, anything that consistently elevates your adrenaline level and puts you in a constant fight-or-flight mode may trigger fibromyalgia. Maybe you can't identify a single significant trigger. Maybe there isn't one. Instead, maybe it was a slow accumulation of many different stressors that, in combination with your genetic predisposition to elevated adrenaline levels, finally triggered fibromyalgia.

After you are reasonably certain you know when the fibromyalgia started and what the potential triggers were, you can start working on your time line of subsequent events and changes in your health. Significant events or changes in your health during the intervening years might help provide clues as to what can help you break the fibromyalgia cycle. For example, as you think about your history, do you remember times when you felt better? If so, what was different in your life? If you can determine when you felt better and why, you'll know what you need to change.

Use the sample chart on the following pages as a model, and be sure to include spaces for dates, symptoms, life events, stress level, sleep quality, medical treatments, and activity level. The more detail you put into your case history now, the more helpful it will be later. However, the important thing is that you actually create a case history. If you need to start with something very simple and fill in the details later, that is still preferable to putting it off because it seems like an overwhelming and perhaps depressing task. Putting the history of your illness on paper will help clear up a lot of the confusion about why your symptoms vary as they do and will help reveal hidden patterns. Depending on how long you've had fibromyalgia, you may want to categorize your case history by month or by year. Once you start working toward recovery, you'll want to update your chart on a weekly basis.

Completing your case history may be emotionally difficult. Human beings are truly resilient and can endure a great amount of pain and suffering. However, our brain also tends to help us forget just how bad things were. When you start delving into your past, you may come across some painful memories and experiences that you would rather not remember. You are a very strong person to have endured all you have and still be looking for help. I know that you want nothing more than to leave the past behind, to move forward, and to get on with your life. The past, however, is an important component of fibromyalgia, and I urge you to complete this exercise, even if parts of it are difficult. Take a look at the following sample history:

CASE HISTORY: SAMPLE CHART/TIME LINE

ORIGINAL SYMPTOMS: pain in back, neck, arms, terrible allergies, asthma

DATE FIRST NOTICED: March 2004

POTENTIAL CAUSES: prolonged arm pain, separation from husband, insomnia, overwork, extended illness

Dates	Symptoms	Life Events	Stress Level	Sleep Quality	Medical Treatments	Activity Level (1–10)
March–April 2004	Painful wrists, forearms, hips. Find typing difficult. Pain in lower back while kayaking. Terrible allergies.	Separated from husband. Working overtime in the office. Great times with friends, but also extreme sadness. 2 new housemates move in.	High	Terrible due to stress	Osteopathic manipulation Ice Counseling Ambien (zolpidem) for sleep Lost 15 lb in 3 months. Not previously overweight.	9 Still running every weekend. Working 12-hour days or more.
May	Same	Working on marriage with husband. Extremely busy at work. Vacation at end of May.	High	Poor	Same as above. Developed severe illness while on vacation. Used amoxicillin, Zithromax (azithromycin). Trip to ER Memorial Day weekend due to extreme dizziness and weakness. ER doc prescribes prednisone for severe allergies	8 Pain is starting to limit work and play.

Month	Physical symptoms	Activities	Stress	Sleep	Medical	Rating	Function
June	Extreme pain in joints and muscles. Wrists hurt too much to hold a book.	Spending time with husband. Canceled weekend trip due to illness. Extremely busy preparing for big presentation at work.	Extremely high	Very poor—difficulty sleeping due to stress and now also pain	Saw allergist. Diagnosed with tendonitis in wrists and arms. Started physical therapy. More antibiotics for infection.	6	All of my energy goes into work. No energy left for any fun activities. Too much pain.
July	Tremendous pain in muscles and joints. Driving is difficult. Extreme exhaustion. Unable to lift even a cup of water. Allergies are unbearable. Asthma develops.	Weekend trip with husband. Relationship improving. Too tired for much fun. Unable to work.	High A lot of stress over how sick I am.	Same as above	Continued PT—no improvement. Doctor prescribes Advair (fluticasone and salmeterol) for asthma, Nexium (esomeprazole) for acid reflux, and Vioxx (rofecoxib) for arm pain.	3	Unable to engage in any normal activities. Some walking.

(Continued)

CASE HISTORY: SAMPLE CHART/TIME LINE (Continued)

Dates	Symptoms	Life Events	Stress Level	Sleep Quality	Medical Treatments	Activity Level (1–10)
August	Same as above. Asthma comes and goes, which I've never had before. Extremely depressed from pain. Crying all the time.	Attend marriage workshop with husband. Decide to move back in together.	High Stressed about pain and inability to work.	Unable to exercise, which makes it increasingly difficult to sleep	Trigger-point injections Switch to a different physical therapist.	3 Same as above
September	Pain level in wrists and arms goes down. Increase in energy.	Husband moves back in. Celebrate anniversary.	Moderate	Improved	Tried acupuncture. Still treating allergies. New sleep medication.	3 Hire housekeeper, as I can't do it.

Even though this history only covers a few months, I can still learn a lot about this patient. There are certainly enough triggers for this patient to have developed fibromyalgia. She indicates a separation from her husband, a demanding work schedule, pain in her body from working too much, and a consistently high stress level. She has trouble sleeping and also experienced a difficult illness during this period. Just looking at her chart, I can tell that she's probably a type-A personality who expects a lot from herself. People with this personality type are generally more susceptible to fibromyalgia because they approach everything with such intensity. She probably had tendonitis long before it was diagnosed in June. It seems likely that she entered the fibromyalgia cycle toward the end of May, at the same time she found herself in an emergency room. Things went rapidly downhill from there.

Her underlying medical condition, tendonitis in both arms, became completely unbearable once she began to experience amplified pain sensations. Fibromyalgia also heightened her sensitivity with regard to allergies, and she developed asthma for the first time ever. As her activity level plummeted and her pain increased, she became depressed, and understandably so. The initial event that created excessive stress in her life was resolved once she and her husband reconciled. The fibromyalgia continued because her original symptom, pain, became the primary trigger. She also developed depression, which feeds into the vicious cycle of fibromyalgia. Her problems with sleep had started in response to marital problems. Even though her stress level was reduced by August, the pain now made it impossible to sleep.

This patient's history only made sense once she documented it in a chronological fashion. Until that point, her symptoms and problems were an overwhelming blur of pain, confusion, and exhaustion. Once I showed her how the triggers and symptoms matched the predictable cycle of fibromyalgia, we were able to develop an extremely effective treatment program for her. Now it's your turn.

Fibromyalgia Triggers

Once you have completed your case history, check to see if any of the following fibromyalgia triggers are on your chart:

_____ Poor, interrupted, or nonrefreshing sleep (1)

_____ Sleep apnea (2)

_____ Stress (1)

_____ Anxiety and/or panic disorder (2)

_____ Depression (2)

_____ Posttraumatic stress disorder (2)

_____ Bipolar disorder/manic depression (2)

_____ Schizophrenia/other serious psychiatric disorder (2)

_____ Severe osteoarthritis/painful inflammatory disease, other chronic painful disorders (2)

_____ Painful trauma, such as from a car accident (2)

_____ Restless legs syndrome (1)

_____ Hypermobility (double jointedness) (1)

Add up the numbers associated with each of the triggers you checked off. Do you have more than three points? If so, you have enough triggers to consider the possibility of fibromyalgia.

Fibromyalgia Symptoms

Place a check mark next to any of the following symptoms on your list:

_____ Widespread, variable aches and pains

_____ Noninflammatory pain that doesn't respond to medication

_____ Fatigue

_____ Morning stiffness

_____ Restless sleep

_____ Increased sensitivity to allergens

_____ Confusion or difficulty concentrating

_____ Easily irritated skin

_____ Numbness

_____ Itching

_____ Feeling too cold or too hot

_____ Sensitivity to bright lights or loud noises

_____ Intense tastes or smells

_____ Skin that readily flushes

_____ Discomfort in a crowded environment

Do your symptoms vary as the causes noted in the first list intensify or improve? For example, do you tend to experience more pain and fatigue whenever your stress level is particularly high? Or, conversely, do you find you have more energy and suffer from less pain whenever you're able to get more sleep and avoid many of your normal stressors?

Do You Have Fibromyalgia?

If your triggers add up to three points and your symptoms vary with these triggers, then you have fibromyalgia. It is very important to note that the symptoms must vary with the triggers in order to confirm a fibromyalgia diagnosis. If your symptoms are stable and do not vary with your particular fibromyalgia triggers, then it is highly unlikely that you have fibromyalgia. Of course, if you have severe fibromyalgia, it may seem as if your symptoms never let up. This is why creating a case history is so important. At some point in the fibromyalgia cycle, you should be able to identify a time when your symptoms varied in step with the triggers.

If I Don't Have Any of the Triggers, Can I Still Have Fibromyalgia?

If you haven't experienced any of the triggers listed above, you probably don't have fibromyalgia. However, there are still three possibilities.

1. You may have one of the causes of fibromyalgia that's difficult for you to detect, such as lupus or sleep apnea. I have often found fibromyalgia to be the symptom that ultimately leads to a diagnosis of lupus.
2. There may be something else—a serious disease, perhaps—that's showing up in the form of pain and fatigue. If you're suffering from a serious disease that has not yet been detected, there's really no time to waste in seeking out proper assessment and treatment.

3. Something may be interfering with your ability to properly assess what your body is experiencing. For example, if you have posttraumatic stress disorder (PTSD), you may not have healed as thoroughly as you think you have. That is, you may think you've put it all behind you, but your adrenaline system is still inclined to elevate readily. Are you one of these people? Pause a moment to ask yourself this: Do you feel as though your adrenaline level is often too high? Do you feel on edge? Are you easily startled? Do you tend to show anger or defensiveness more than those around you? Have you ever experienced road rage? Do your legs jerk at night? Do you have trouble sleeping? If so, then you may still suffer from the lingering effects of PTSD.

It is safe to rule out fibromyalgia as a diagnosis if you can not find any causes, including such hidden triggers as sleep apnea, or if you are diagnosed with another medical condition that fully explains your symptoms.

Checking for Other Medical Conditions

As I discussed earlier, fibromyalgia used to be considered a cop-out diagnosis. That is, doctors pulled out this diagnosis when they couldn't find anything else wrong with you. This line of thinking is flawed for two reasons. First, even if you are diagnosed with another painful illness or disease, you shouldn't rule out fibromyalgia. Second, if you are diagnosed with fibromyalgia, you can still have other medical conditions contributing to your symptoms. At this point, you probably know whether you have fibromyalgia. Regardless of your conclusion, you need to work with a healthcare provider to determine whether you might have rheumatoid arthritis, lupus, polymyalgia rheumatica (inflammation of the hips and shoulders), hypothyroidism, other endocrine disorders, or peripheral neuropathy. These are conditions that are either closely associated with fibromyalgia or have similar signs and symptoms to those seen in fibromyalgia. Most of these conditions can be tested for with a physical examination, laboratory tests, X-rays, or a nerve conduction test.

Going After the Triggers

In the world of fibromyalgia, the focus has always been on treating the symptoms, such as pain and depression, because the cause of the illness itself was unknown. Treating symptoms is actually an important component of treating fibromyalgia, as you have seen or even experienced how easy it is for symptoms to become triggers. If you have fibromyalgia and have taken the time to complete your case history and identify your triggers, you have taken an important step toward breaking the cycle of fibromyalgia. Working on your triggers is the single best way to treat your fibromyalgia. Go directly after the root of all your other problems—namely, your elevated fight-or-flight response. Whenever you begin to make changes to reduce your fight-or-flight response, your brain will begin to rebuild its dopamine reserves, even if they've been severely depleted. Review your list of triggers, and make notes on what actions you can take to resolve them. Some triggers may be physical in nature and require surgery or other medical treatments. Other causes may be psychological in nature and require a different treatment approach.

You should work closely with your doctor to resolve any other medical conditions you might have. Your body has an impressive array of defenses against illness, disease, and injury. When something goes wrong, the body is always trying to heal itself. Fibromyalgia completely overwhelms this system of defenses. Fibromyalgia literally feeds off the other weaknesses in your body. Every sensation perceived as amplified by fibromyalgia comes from something that's actually happening in your body. Your ANS has simply lost its ability to filter sensations, so you feel them more than you normally would. If the original painful sensation can be reduced, then the amplified signal your brain ultimately experiences is less likely to cause you as much distress. This applies to every sensation, not just to aches and pains. Fibromyalgia is so overwhelming that people sometimes ignore problems that don't seem as severe. You can't afford to do that. Your body needs to be as strong as possible. If you can take steps to help your body recover from other problems, even if they seem trivial in comparison, you will have additional strength for your fight against fibromyalgia.

Keep in mind that even the most diligent work to resolve your triggers is not going to yield a quick fix. It's hard to take action if you are fatigued and in pain. This is why in part 2 of this book, I will first explain how to get some immediate relief. Once things calm down, you can make a thorough, long-term plan to finally rein in your overactive fight-or-flight response. If this seems impossible right now, let me tell you that I did it. Hundreds of patients have done this until they had no fibromyalgia symptoms at all. Even if you have had pain for decades, you were not born with fibromyalgia. However, you may have to make some drastic changes and face difficult decisions. The one thing I can provide here is a definitive guide to what needs to be done and how to do it. The second part of this book will use the science of fibromyalgia to provide you with a definitive recovery plan. Please join me and a growing number of patients around the country in taking back your life!

In a Nutshell . . .

- The diagnostic criteria currently used by doctors to diagnose fibromyalgia rely on outdated material and inaccurate assumptions. Many people are misdiagnosed.
- The current diagnostic criteria make it impossible to catch fibromyalgia in the early stages. *You* are in the best position to catch fibromyalgia at the beginning of the cycle.
- Develop a detailed case history, and determine your initial and subsequent fibromyalgia triggers. Compare your triggers and symptoms with my diagnostic criteria.
- If you have enough of the fibromyalgia triggers and your symptoms vary in step with these triggers, there is a good chance you have fibromyalgia.
- Work with a doctor to confirm your diagnosis, and check for other medical conditions that may be responsible for your symptoms. Doctors routinely test for rheumatoid arthritis, lupus, hypothyroidism, and other problems that cause similar symptoms.
- If you do have fibromyalgia, take steps to resolve any other medical conditions contributing to your symptoms.

PART II

Recovering from Fibromyalgia

Moving Beyond Fibromyalgia

You can only recover from fibromyalgia by recognizing and resolving the triggers that are keeping your fight-or-flight response on high alert. You are essentially rebalancing your autonomic nervous system, which for too long has been tipped toward a state of fight-or-flight. Once you rein in your fight-or-flight response, your body will have the opportunity to replenish your critically low levels of dopamine. As balance is restored, the hypersensitivity that characterizes fibromyalgia will disappear and you can once again enjoy the day-to-day pleasures of simply being alive and pain-free. The question is, what's the best path for your recovery?

Develop a Long-Term Recovery Plan

In order to develop your recovery plan, review the case history you developed in chapter 5. If you have not completed this task, it's time to put pen to paper. Otherwise, you may come away from this book feeling inspired but overwhelmed. The three most important steps to recovery are to (1) restore your sleep cycle, (2) reduce stress by controlling your fight-or-flight response, and (3) identify and resolve underlying medical and physical causes. Going right to work on these fibromyalgia triggers is always my preferred treatment option.

Each chapter in part 2 covers important information on the best ways to help your body heal from months, years, or even decades of suffering from fibromyalgia. While some of these chapters address the key fibromyalgia triggers, such as stress and sleep disorders, other chapters focus on effective ways to reduce symptoms through dietary changes, prescription medications, exercise, and such complementary therapies as massage. As you read each chapter in part 2, start developing a recovery plan tailored to your specific needs. With each chapter, write down specific steps you can take to help reverse the fibromyalgia cycle. When you have finished the book, you will have a concrete set of steps you can follow to restore your health. No matter how many steps are on your list, don't feel intimidated by the road to recovery. The trick is to start small and choose some initial steps that will be easy to accomplish. If you try to make too many changes at once, it will be hard to know which particular changes are actually making a difference.

While the first few chapters in part 2 focus on important lifestyle changes (and I recommend implementing these first), it may be that your symptoms are so severe that you will not be able to tackle these without the aid of short-term prescription medications. If that is the case, chapter 10 discusses some prescription medication options in detail. As you feel better and accomplish the early objectives of your plan, you will find that you can take on more challenging goals. If you have setbacks, don't give up or feel frustrated. Give your body the time and space it needs to start healing. It is far better to make slow, steady progress than to take on too much, get frustrated, and then give up.

As you address underlying medical causes and follow the recommendations related to sleep, stress, diet, prescription medications, exercise, and complementary therapies, your symptoms will improve and then ultimately disappear as you successfully resolve your fibromyalgia triggers. Once you have recovered from fibromyalgia, you may find that you are actually healthier than ever before, thanks to some of the lifestyle changes you will make along the way. When you are symptom-free, continue to follow the key elements of your recovery plan for another six to eight months to ensure that your dopamine levels have stabilized. After that, you will no longer need to follow a specific plan for staying fibromyalgia-free. However, you should keep in mind that a healthy mind and body are your best defense against developing fibromyalgia again.

Commit to Recovery

Following your recovery plan will take dedication, commitment, and planning. Starting with just one month, make your health a priority. You owe it to yourself. If you have a job, see if you can take some time off from work or at least reduce your hours. If you have a family, find someone to help you with some of those responsibilities. These may seem like difficult and even selfish decisions, but if you give yourself a little time now, everyone will benefit in the future, when you start feeling better.

Now that you know more about fibromyalgia, take the time to talk to your family and friends about your condition. Explain to them what is really happening in your body and why your symptoms vary the way they do. Like you, they will be greatly relieved to know that there is a solution to your problem. Let them know that you will need their support and encouragement in order to succeed in escaping the misery of fibromyalgia. If you can, find someone who is willing to discuss your progress with you on a weekly basis. There are times when this process will be difficult, and you will need consistent moral support.

Create a Progress Journal

In order to track your progress, you will need to create a Progress Journal. Use your Progress Journal to record your case history, develop your recovery plan, write down your personal goals, and track any changes in your symptoms. Your Progress Journal will help you determine whether specific changes, such as trying a new type of exercise or a different medication, are making a difference in how you feel. To create your Progress Journal, simply purchase a spiral notebook and keep a chronological record of any changes you make and how you feel each day. It's always a good idea to specifically note the quality of your sleep, your stress level, and any symptoms you experience during the day. Your Progress Journal will be an important tool as you assess whether specific steps you take are having an effect on how you feel. It will also help your physician determine whether any medications you take need to be modified or changed.

Another good way to track your progress is to make a list of the things you would like to do but can't because of fibromyalgia. For example, perhaps you wish you could sit through a movie without being uncomfortable the entire time. Or perhaps you would like to weed your garden again. What about waking up in the morning without being stiff? Write down small goals, medium goals, and super-size goals in the front of your Progress Journal. Each month, use these goals to measure your progress. You'll be amazed at the deep satisfaction you'll find in accomplishing even the simplest of activities without pain. Although it is hard to imagine, the misery of fibromyalgia serves to intensify the sweetness and joy of simply being alive as you start to reclaim your life.

CHAPTER 6

Sleeping Well

An incessant buzzing breaks the morning silence. Lisa hits the snooze button with more force than necessary to silence the intrusive sound. Is it possible, she wonders, to be more exhausted this morning than she was last night? Lisa doesn't remember waking up during the night, but she doesn't feel as if she got much sleep, either. The disheveled state of her bed linens confirms that her sleep was restless. As is the case with over 90 percent of the patients I see, one of the most important factors keeping Lisa trapped in the fibromyalgia cycle is a consistent lack of deep, restorative sleep. You have probably noticed that your pain and other symptoms are directly affected by the amount and quality of sleep you get at night. After a few nights of good sleep, you start feeling a little bit better. On the other hand, a few nights of really poor sleep exacerbate your symptoms. Providing for improved sleep will immediately help you get the upper hand in the battle against fibromyalgia. Improving your sleep is so important that it is the first step you should take on your journey toward recovery. In this chapter, you'll learn about the relationship between poor sleep and fibromyalgia and the common sleep disorders associated with fibromyalgia. Most important, you'll learn what you can do to improve the quality of your sleep immediately.

Placing a Priority on Sleep

A critical step toward recovery is making improved sleep a priority in your life. In addition to increases in pain, a lack of quality sleep impairs such cognitive functions as memory and decision-making skills, exacerbating the frustration of fibro fog. Poor sleep contributes to fatigue, mood swings, and symptoms of depression. You may have suffered from sleep problems for years, or they may have developed in association with the onset of fibromyalgia. Regardless, there are concrete steps you can take to improve your sleep immediately. Increasing the quality of your sleep will produce some of the most immediate and dramatic effects of any step you take toward recovery.

As sleep improves, your body's sorely needed but diminished supply of dopamine will have a chance to catch up with the demands of your overactive fight-or-flight response. Improved sleep won't totally solve the dopamine problem, but most people feel positive results after a few weeks of it. Consistently sleeping well will also improve your mental clarity, reduce your fatigue, and provide a big boost to your immune system. Consequently, you'll have more energy to take the other steps toward recovery described in this book.

Many of the new patients who come into my office inform me that improving their sleep is a lost cause. They tell me that they've tried everything, and they still can't sleep. On the other end of the spectrum, some people aren't even aware that they have a problem with sleep. Don't give up on sleep! Sleep researchers have recently made discoveries regarding the best ways to approach insomnia and other sleep problems. No matter what you've tried in the past, you owe it to yourself to try another approach to sleeping well. You simply can't afford to ignore this step. Let's start with understanding more about why you don't sleep well.

The Relationship Between Poor Sleep and Fibromyalgia

Although a sleepless night may seem incredibly lonely, you are far from alone in your inability to hit the sack and be out like a light. There are many reasons that people have trouble sleeping. In fact, sleep researchers have categorized over seventy types of sleep disorders! The most familiar of these is insomnia—a problem most people deal with at some point in their lives. According to the National Sleep Foundation's 2002 Sleep in America poll, 58 percent of adults experience symptoms of insomnia a few nights a week or more. The National Institutes of Health estimates that seventy million Americans suffer from a sleep disorder. These figures are staggering, considering the importance of sleep to our physical and mental health. Anyone with a chronic sleep disorder is automatically at greater risk of developing fibromyalgia, and virtually everyone with fibromyalgia has a sleep disorder. Let's explore the relationship between the two problems a little more closely.

Although a sleep disorder such as sleep apnea can be the primary cause of fibromyalgia, it is usually poor sleep in combination with another trigger that causes the disorder. Regardless of your prefibromyalgia sleep patterns, your natural sleep cycle will quickly deteriorate with the onset of fibromyalgia. In a normal sleep/wake cycle, the activity level of the sympathetic nervous system decreases at night so that you can relax and go to sleep. As we've discussed, an overactive sympathetic nervous system inhibits sleep, interrupting your natural circadian rhythm. Even if you do fall asleep at night, chances are that your nervous system interferes with the natural progression of sleep during the night.

A normal sleep cycle has five phases: stages 1 to 4 and rapid eye movement (REM) sleep. During the night, the body progresses through each of these stages, with REM sleep, also known as dream sleep, being the final stage. After the body achieves REM sleep, the cycle starts over with stage 1 sleep. The complete sleep cycle averages 90 to 110 minutes and may repeat six or more times during the night. Stage 1 sleep is very light, and if awakened, you may not realize that you were sleeping. In stage 2 sleep, your brain waves start slowing down in preparation for stages 3 and 4. In stage 3 sleep, the brain begins producing extremely slow brain waves known as delta waves that are periodically interrupted by faster waves known as alpha waves. In normal stage 4 sleep, the brain waves are almost entirely delta waves. Many of the body's restorative functions take place during the deepest stages of sleep, including the replenishment of dopamine, antibodies, growth hormone, and other important substances. Fibromyalgia patients suffer from an insufficient amount of the deep, restorative sleep that takes place in stages 3 and 4. The final stage in the sleep cycle is REM sleep. Following REM sleep, the cycle repeats, and as the night progresses, less and less time is spent in deep sleep. After a normal night of sleep, the body should be done with stage 3 and 4 sleep before the alarm clock ever goes off.

In 1974, Dr. Harvey Moldofsky of the Clarke Institute of Psychiatry in Toronto, Canada, published a landmark study that showed how pain could be induced by interrupting stages 3 and 4 sleep. Dr. Moldofsky hired healthy students, aged nineteen to twenty-five, and deprived six of them of stage 4 sleep and seven of them of REM sleep. This was done for three consecutive nights. The subjects whose stage 4 sleep had been interrupted began showing signs of fibromyalgia. This wasn't the case for the subjects who had been denied REM sleep. In addition, the students who had been deprived of stage 4 sleep began to experience overwhelming tiredness and loss of appetite, and one even suffered from nausea and diarrhea. Once sleep was restored to normal for these subjects, all of their fibromyalgia-like symptoms disappeared.

More recent sleep studies show that alpha-wave activity, normally limited to the early stages of sleep, often continues unabated in fibromyalgia patients. This alpha-wave intrusion interrupts the sleep cycle, either preventing them from achieving stage 3 or 4 sleep or greatly decreasing the restorative qualities of these sleep stages. Alpha-wave intrusions account for the frequent awakening and restless activity that characterize nonrestorative sleep. Alpha-wave intrusions during delta-wave sleep are far more prevalent in people with fibromyalgia. In a 2001 study conducted at Federal University of São Paulo in Brazil, 70 percent of fibromyalgia patients showed increased alpha-wave activity as compared to only 26 percent of participants without fibromyalgia.

Even in healthy people, the impact of alpha-wave intrusions is unrefreshing sleep, diffuse muscle pain, tenderness, and fatigue. Given the heightened sensitivity that accompanies fibromyalgia, the impact of continually interrupted sleep can have devastating consequences. A 1996 study at the University of Connecticut School of Medicine enlisted fifty women with fibromyalgia to record their sleep quality, pain intensity, and attention to pain for thirty days. Researchers discovered that the women consistently reported increased pain intensity following a poor night of sleep. A more sophisticated study conducted in 2001 by Dr. Moldofsky compared increased alpha-wave activity in fibromyalgia patients with increases in pain and in the number of tender points. All the patients who experienced an overlap of alpha- and delta-wave activity reported a worsening of pain after sleep. Ninety percent of these patients also experienced an increase in the number of tender points.

Sleep Disorders Associated with Fibromyalgia

The three sleep disorders most closely associated with fibromyalgia are chronic insomnia, sleep apnea, and restless legs syndrome. You may suffer from one or more of these conditions. As you read through the common causes of insomnia, use your Progress Journal to make a list of what keeps you up at night and the steps you can take to resolve these problems.

Chronic Insomnia

Insomnia is not an illness but a symptom that something else is wrong. Almost everyone experiences occasional insomnia as a result of stress, illness, travel, or other circumstances. My patients generally find sleep difficult because of an overactive mind and an uncomfortable body. Does your mind race when you lie down at night? Do you find yourself reviewing everything that happened during the day, often focusing on things that went wrong? Are you worried about what will happen tomorrow or later this week? Are you replaying an argument in your head, trying to figure out what you could have said differently? Are you using the bedroom to make battle plans for tomorrow? Maybe you're worrying that you're not going to get enough sleep—again.

Any of these thoughts can prompt the fight-or-flight response to spring into action, pumping up the sympathetic nervous system just when it should be shutting down. With fibromyalgia, your fight-or-flight response is already on a hair trigger, just waiting for a cue from the brain to dispense more stress hormones into your bloodstream. When your mind starts racing at night, that's the only signal it needs to turn up the volume, making sleep all but impossible.

During stage 1 sleep, you may experience a series of body jerks powerful enough to wake you up. Although it can be normal for the body to twitch as it falls asleep, the increased activity of the sympathetic nervous system likely exacerbates these twitches until they are strong enough to inhibit sleep. These involuntary muscle contractions are designed to keep you awake and alert. Your overactive fight-or-flight response is doing its very best to keep you from "letting your guard down" in spite of your exhaustion.

Pain also inhibits sleep by triggering the fight-or-flight response. It's very challenging to fall asleep if your body is aching and your joints are painful. You may succeed in tuning out some of your pain during the day by keeping your mind focused on other things. However, when you lie down at night, you are finally alone with your pain, and your brain can't ignore it anymore. As you toss and turn, trying to find a comfortable position, your frustration increases and your mind kicks into action. Maybe you start thinking about the fact that you really need to sleep but you know you won't be able to. Together, a painful body and a restless mind present a powerful barrier to sleep.

Other underlying conditions can cause or contribute to insomnia, including indigestion, acid reflux, allergies or nasal congestion, hyperthyroidism, menopause, anxiety, depression, nausea, and bladder problems. A lack of exercise may also have a great impact on how well you sleep. If you have an inconsistent sleep schedule due to a job or a tendency to nap during the day, this will further disrupt your natural circadian rhythm. Caffeine, alcohol, and nicotine also interfere with your ability to sleep soundly.

Finally, jobs that require you to work night shifts—or worse yet, involve varying shifts—should be avoided. People need regular and predictable sleep schedules, so it's no surprise that shift work has often been found to worsen fibromyalgia. This also applies to patients who travel frequently for work, especially if that involves changing time zones.

If you suffer from insomnia, there are two ways to improve sleep: change your habits and attitudes as they relate to sleep and take prescription or over-the-counter medications. Recent studies have shown that behavioral changes or behavioral changes in combination with medication are the most effective cures for insomnia. In these studies, the participants who made only behavioral changes were the most likely to remain normal sleepers during an extended follow-up period. This approach has also been specifically studied in fibromyalgia patients, with very encouraging results. However, you should not expect your sleep patterns to completely normalize until you have successfully resolved any other fibromyalgia triggers that are keeping your fight-or-flight response on high alert.

Sleep Apnea

If you think you sleep well but awaken tired or you know you snore, the first step is to investigate whether you have sleep apnea. Sleep apnea, a temporary cessation of breathing, usually occurs in association with fat buildup or the loss of muscle tone in the neck associated with aging. These changes allow the windpipe to collapse during breathing, when muscles relax during sleep. The collapsed windpipe blocks air flow for ten seconds to a minute, leaving the sleeping person struggling to breathe. When the person's blood oxygen level falls, the brain responds by waking the person enough to tighten the upper airway muscles and open the windpipe. The person may snort or gasp and then return to sleep without any conscious memory of nearly suffocating. This may happen hundreds of times each night! An estimated eighteen million Americans suffer from sleep apnea, with the majority of these cases remaining undiagnosed.

Sleep apnea is commonly associated with snoring, obesity, and daytime fatigue. Even subtle cases of sleep apnea can trigger your fight-or-flight response. Each time your oxygen level falls, the body is faced with a truly life-threatening situation. These constant sleep interruptions also prohibit you from ever reaching the deepest stages of sleep. This is why it's extremely difficult to make headway against fibromyalgia when even a mild case of sleep apnea remains untreated. Sleep apnea can also lead to weight gain, obesity, headaches, high blood pressure, and a host of other health problems. While combating fibromyalgia should probably be a strong enough argument in its own right, there also are many other reasons for aggressively treating sleep apnea.

If you suspect that sleep apnea may be a problem, your doctor can refer you to a sleep center that is equipped to diagnose it. If it turns out that you do have sleep apnea, there are different options for treatment, depending on the severity of your condition. For mild sleep apnea, weight loss or a change in sleeping positions may resolve the problem. For more severe cases, you may need to wear a breathing aid known as a CPAP (continuous positive airway pressure) device. If you've already been diagnosed with sleep apnea but have found it difficult to use a CPAP device, you should try again. It can take months to get used to wearing a nasal mask, but it may prove to be well worth the effort. There also are a number of other options for treating sleep apnea, some of which are surgical. If you continue to have problems with sleep apnea, I recommend that you talk to your doctor about different treatment options.

Restless Legs Syndrome

Over 30 percent of people with fibromyalgia also suffer from restless legs syndrome (RLS), an unpleasant sensation in the legs that is only alleviated by movement. Like fibromyalgia, RLS is linked to an imbalance in the autonomic nervous system. The symptoms of RLS are often worse when a person is sitting down or lying in bed, trying to sleep. RLS is most common among the elderly, but it can occur at any age. Fortunately, it can be alleviated with medication. Medications commonly used for the treatment of RLS include Requip (ropinirole), Mirapex (pramipexole), Sinemet (carbidopa and levodopa), and Permax (pergolide). As I mentioned in part 1, Dr. Andrew Holman's recognition of the overlap between RLS and fibromyalgia led to new discoveries about the origins of fibromyalgia. RLS patients benefit from lower doses of one of the same dopamine-enhancing medications (Mirapex and Requip) that help alleviate fibromyalgia symptoms at much higher doses. If you have RLS, ask your doctor about taking Requip to calm your restless limbs.

Getting a Good Night's Sleep

Resolving sleep problems can be challenging, and you may have already tried to improve your sleep without success. Now that you understand the relationship between poor sleep and fibromyalgia, you should have sufficient motivation to try again. The following principles will help improve the quality of your sleep.

Change Your Attitude About Sleep

If you have chronic insomnia, you probably don't have a very positive attitude about sleep. It's common for insomniacs to worry extensively about how much sleep they're getting and the potential impacts of a poor night of sleep. You probably find yourself thinking thoughts like these:

"If I don't get enough sleep tonight, I'm going to feel terrible tomorrow."

"It's been such a stressful day—I know I'm never going to fall asleep tonight."

"It's already too late to get eight hours of sleep."

These thoughts are normal for poor sleepers, but are also very detrimental. In *Say Good Night to Insomnia,* the sleep expert Dr. Gregg Jacobs describes these as negative sleep thoughts. They occur, he explains, almost automatically as a knee-jerk reaction based on your past experiences with sleep. These negative thoughts set you up to fail, as your fears about not sleeping are a powerful trigger of the fight-or-flight response—one that happens at the very moment you are trying to relax enough to sleep. These negative sleep thoughts are also often based on inaccurate assumptions about how much sleep you need and the amount of sleep you probably actually get. Compare the following facts about sleep with your negative thoughts about sleep:

Do you get stressed about not getting eight hours of sleep? The amount of sleep needed by an adult ranges from five to ten hours of sleep a night. The amount of core sleep needed is actually only three to five hours a night. Core sleep is the deepest, most restorative sleep you get during the night. This generally takes place in the earliest hours of sleep. No matter when you fall asleep, chances are, you are still getting some or all of the essential core sleep. Research has shown that people can function normally on less sleep than they think they need.

Instead of worrying about getting eight hours of sleep, focus on being thankful for the core sleep you do get.

Do you spend a lot of time thinking about how much sleep you didn't get? Your perception of how much you slept the previous night is not always accurate. Many times, people will drift into light sleep for a period of time and then wake up and not realize they were actually asleep. This can often happen in the middle of the night. You wake up briefly and glance at the clock. Without realizing it, you fall asleep again and then awaken once more. After a few minutes, you look at the clock and think you have been awake for much longer than is actually the case. *Start making the assumption that you are actually getting more sleep than you think.*

Are you worried about waking up once you fall asleep? Earlier in this chapter, I described how the sleep cycle repeats throughout the night. It's entirely normal for adults to wake up multiple times as they progress through the different stages of sleep. Many times, people are not aware of this happening. If you wake up and then start worrying about the fact that you are awake, your concern will make it more difficult to return to sleep. *If you wake up during the night, reassure yourself that this is a normal part of the sleep cycle.*

You should also keep in mind that the body is very good at making up for lost time. If you sleep poorly one night, you will sleep more deeply the next night, even if you don't sleep all night long. It takes less sleep than you might think to recover from a few nights or even a week of poor sleep. Rather than letting your anxiety about sleep compound your sleep problems, give your body the benefit of the doubt. You are probably getting more sleep than you think. If you can reprogram your mind to have a positive attitude about sleep, you'll increase both the quality and quantity of your sleep. The next time you catch yourself thinking or saying, "I'm never going to sleep tonight!" repress that thought and instead say out loud, "I'm sure I'll get enough sleep tonight. I always get more than I think I'm going to." You'll be amazed at the power of this technique over time.

Change Your Behavior to Improve Sleep

Sleep experts refer to behaviors that influence sleep as sleep hygiene. In the same way that good dental hygiene helps provide for healthy teeth, good sleep hygiene helps provide for a good night's sleep. Many insomniacs lay in bed for hours, determined to fall asleep, too tired to get up, and thoroughly frustrated at their inability to fall asleep. Sound familiar? The problem with this scenario is that they are not actually improving their chances of sleeping more. Instead, their minds associate the bedroom with frustration and insomnia rather than sleep.

The following steps will help your mind and body associate the bedroom with sleep rather than sleeplessness. In the beginning, some of these changes may seem counterintuitive—but they are proven to decrease the amount of time it takes to fall asleep and increase the amount and quality of the sleep you get each night.

During the day, take the following steps to help ensure sleep at night:

- Get up and go to bed at the same time each and every day—even on weekends! This may be difficult at first, but you want your body to be tired at a reasonable hour. Once you establish a regular rhythm in your sleep pattern, you'll find it will be easier to fall asleep, and you'll also feel better. However, you shouldn't try to go to bed until you're sleepy.

- Don't take naps. This will ensure that you're tired when it's time to go to bed.

- You may not feel like exercising yet, but know that developing an exercise program will ultimately help you sleep better. Once you are exercising again, refrain from exercising at least four hours prior to bedtime.

- Develop sleep rituals. It's important to give your body unmistakable cues that it's time to slow down and sleep. Listen to relaxing music, read something soothing for fifteen minutes, have a cup of herbal tea, or do some relaxation exercises.

- Take a hot bath ninety minutes before bedtime. A hot bath will raise your body temperature, and the subsequent drop in body temperature may leave you feeling sleepy.

- Stay away from caffeine for at least four to six hours prior to bedtime. Caffeine is a stimulant that interferes with your ability to fall asleep. Among the substances to beware of are coffee, tea, cola, cocoa, and chocolate.

- Avoid alcohol within four hours of bedtime. While it may seem at first that alcohol helps you get to sleep, since it slows brain activity, it generally leads to a night of fragmented sleep rather than the deep, restorative sleep your body needs. Nicotine is another stimulant that interferes with sleep. Smokers often wake up too early due to nicotine withdrawal.

- Have a light snack before bed. If your stomach is too empty when you go to bed, hunger could end up interfering with your sleep. However, eating a heavy meal just prior to bedtime is equally likely to interfere.

Once you go to bed, follow these rules religiously:

- Use your bed only for sleeping. Refrain from using your bed to watch television, pay bills, work, or read. What you really want is for your mind to associate your bed with sleeping, so that when you go to bed, your body will know for certain that it's time to sleep.
- Make sure your bed and bedroom are quiet and comfortable. A hot room can be uncomfortable, so a cooler room supplied with enough blankets to keep you warm is recommended. In the event that light in the early morning bothers you, get a blackout shade or wear a slumber mask. If noise bothers you, wear earplugs or make use of a "white noise" machine, such as a fan.
- If you can't fall asleep within twenty minutes, get up and do something tedious until you feel sleepy. This is challenging, but you will increase your chances of falling asleep faster if you don't lie in bed, awake. When you get up, don't expose yourself to bright light, since the light cues your brain that it's time to wake up. Read or simply sit in the dark until you feel yourself nodding off, and then return to bed.
- Use sunlight to set your biological clock. As soon as you get up in the morning, go outside and turn your face to the sun for fifteen minutes. This helps regulate your sleep/wake cycle. Bright lights will have the same effect and are more consistently available than sunlight.

Commit to these guidelines for at least a month to determine whether they are helpful for you. Be sure to track your progress in your Progress Journal as you go. These changes will only work if you consistently follow them for an extended period of time. Although these are changes you should adopt for life, it's often easier to commit to them for a specified period of time in the beginning.

Medications for Sleep

Taking medication to induce sleep is not a permanent solution for several reasons. Most sleep medications are only prescribed for short-term use. Long-term use results in dependency—meaning that you can no longer sleep without the medication. Although this dependency is often physical, it can be psychological as well. Many sleep medications lose their efficacy over time, but people continue to believe that they can't sleep without taking a sleeping pill. This psychological dependence can be as difficult to break as any physical dependence. Sleep medications also have side effects, such as daytime sleepiness, and can interfere with the natural progression of the sleep cycle.

Having said all that, I also believe that in some cases, a short-term prescription for sleep medications may prove extremely useful for people with fibromyalgia. Although studies show that the cognitive-behavioral approach to treating insomnia is superior to the pharmaceutical approach, the people in these studies didn't have severe fibromyalgia. Pain and any associated anxiety about your pain can make it extremely difficult to sleep. An appropriate medication may help restore your sleep long enough for you to rebuild your supply of dopamine. Once your dopamine levels increase, your fibromyalgia symptoms should decrease, and you will be more likely to succeed with the behavioral changes described above.

Resolving sleep issues for fibromyalgia patients requires a long-term solution. If your doctor determines that a short course of sleep medication is needed initially to restore your sleep cycle, you should incorporate the behavioral changes described above simultaneously. This will help ensure a smooth transition once you stop taking medication.

There are several types of medication commonly prescribed for insomnia. Your doctor can make a decision regarding the right type for you based on your current sleep patterns. Some of the most common medications for insomnia are briefly described below. If you try a course of prescription sleeping medications, track the dosage and results in your Progress Journal, as illustrated here. This will help you and your doctor determine the best medication for improving your sleep.

DATE	Oct 15
MEDICATION	Lunesta (eszopiclone)
DOSE	2 mg
FELL ASLEEP EASILY? AT WHAT TIME?	Yes—10:30 pm
NIGHTTIME WAKENINGS?	Twice—briefly
FINAL TIME AWAKE	7:00 am
REFRESHED IN MORNING?	Yes

Sleep medications do not mix well with alcohol. If you decide to take sleep medications, refrain from having an evening drink. People with sleep apnea should never take sleep medications. Many sleep medications are respiratory depressants that may exacerbate sleep apnea.

Prescription Benzodiazepines

Ativan (lorazepam), Xanax (alprazolam), Valium (diazepam), Klonopin (clonazepam), and Halcion (triazolam) belong to a family of hypnotic medications known as benzodiazepines. Commonly prescribed for insomnia, these drugs are safe and effective sleep medications to use for short periods of time. Unfortunately, benzodiazepines have some unpleasant side effects. Many of these drugs have an extended half-life, meaning they stay in your system longer than is needed for sleep and therefore may result in daytime sleepiness. These drugs can also cause rebound insomnia when you stop taking them, temporarily making it even harder to sleep. People can also develop a tolerance to these drugs in as little as two weeks, negating any sedating effect they may have. In order to reduce the occurrence of these problems, avoid taking medication every night. When you are ready to stop taking medication, break your pills in half, and taper off gradually. This will help prevent rebound insomnia.

Another problem with these drugs is that they reduce both REM sleep and delta-wave sleep. Delta-wave sleep, as you'll remember, is the type of sleep that fibromyalgia patients already have trouble getting enough of.

Prescription Non-benzodiazepines

In recent years, other drugs have been developed that help people achieve sleep without the drawbacks of benzodiazepines. The downside is that these medications can be much more expensive.

Ambien (zolpidem) may be one of the best options for the short-term treatment of insomnia. Ambien is rapidly absorbed and helps put you to sleep in less time than most benzodiazepines. It also has a much shorter half-life, allowing you to wake up refreshed, without any "hangover" effects. Ambien has not been shown to cause a rebound effect, and it doesn't interfere with delta-wave sleep.

There are several other new sleep medications on the market, including Sonata (zaleplon) and Lunesta (eszopiclone), which are similar to Ambien in their effectiveness. Like Ambien, Sonata is approved for short-term use (generally seven to ten days). There is some evidence that Ambien may increase the total amount of sleep time, but comparative studies are limited due to the recent appearance of these drugs. Lunesta does not specify a treatment duration, but all prescription sleeping medications are best used for the minimum amount of time necessary. Your doctor should be able to help you determine the most effective sleep aid based on the characteristics of your insomnia.

Over-the-Counter Sleep Medications

The most widely used over-the-counter (OTC) sleep medications are the same drugs found in antihistamines. Anyone who has taken Benadryl (diphenhydramine) for allergies knows that it has an extremely sedating effect. It's no surprise, then, that the active ingredient in Benadryl is identical to the sedating agent found in OTC sleep aids like Tylenol PM. Doxylamine succinate is another antihistamine commonly found in sleep aids, such as Unisom. These drugs can be effective as an occasional remedy for insomnia, but they can also cause a marked "hangover," making it difficult to get out of bed the next day. For some people, these medications may cause anxiety. You should follow the same precautions as you would with prescription sleep aids. These medications should not be taken with alcohol or for extended periods of time. Do not take these medications in combination with any other sleep medication.

Supplements

Many supplements are marketed as "natural" sleep aids. These include melatonin, valerian root, and kava root. Although these substances aren't regulated by the Food and Drug Administration, their potential side effects should be taken just as seriously.

Melatonin is naturally secreted by the body's pineal gland and helps regulate your circadian rhythm. In other countries, including Canada, melatonin is considered a drug, and manufacturers are required to go through an extensive application process before making it available to consumers. In the United States, no similar safeguards exist. The effectiveness of melatonin has not been proven in large-scale clinical trials, and there is no information available regarding risks from long-term use.

Valerian and kava root both have sedating properties and may be useful as an occasional supplement for bedtime relaxation. Valerian and kava have both been implicated in causing liver toxicity and should not be used for extended periods of time. Chamomile tea also has some relaxing qualities and may be a safer choice if you are looking for something to help you relax.

I can't place enough emphasis on the importance of ensuring quality sleep in the fight against fibromyalgia. In the beginning, you should take whatever steps are necessary to ensure that you are benefiting from the restorative effects of sleep. Whatever method you choose in the short term, keep in mind that a long-term solution is needed as well. I think you'll be pleasantly surprised to find out just how effective a behavioral approach is to ensuring a good night's sleep, night after night.

In a Nutshell . . .

- Poor sleep in combination with another trigger causes fibromyalgia.
- In order to recover from fibromyalgia, you must resolve any sleep issues you have.
- Fibromyalgia patients suffer from an insufficient amount of the deep, restorative sleep that takes place in the later stages of the sleep cycle.
- Many of the body's restorative functions happen during the deepest stages of sleep, including the synthesis of dopamine, antibodies, and growth hormone.
- A night of poor sleep is inevitably followed by increased pain, as dopamine is not replenished.
- The most common sleep disorders associated with fibromyalgia are insomnia, sleep apnea, and restless legs syndrome.
- Sleep apnea and restless legs syndrome can be successfully treated with medications and other medical interventions. See your doctor if you suffer from these conditions.
- Behavioral changes are the most effective way to resolve insomnia over the long term.
- In some situations, a short-term course of sleep medication may be necessary to improve sleep.
- Over-the-counter sleep medications and sleep supplements should be used sparingly and with the same precautions taken with prescription sleep medications.
- As your sleep improves, your diminished supply of dopamine will have a chance to catch up with the demands of your overactive fight-or-flight response. As your dopamine levels increase, you'll start feeling better.

CHAPTER 7

Reducing Stress: Easier Said Than Done

Simply put, alleviating stress is the solution to recovering from fibromyalgia. This chapter will teach you how to reduce the pervasive stress that is the hallmark of the modern world. Rather than encouraging you to put your entire life on hold, I'll teach you how to take control of your fight-or-flight response and reduce the demands on a revved-up sympathetic nervous system. Included in this chapter are straightforward steps for reducing stress that you can implement immediately. If you take them seriously, you're likely to experience tangible results within a month. Over the long term, your entire life will flow more smoothly, and you'll reap all the health benefits of a life without elevated stress levels. In the event that you struggle with more severe psychological issues such as depression, I'll also offer some suggestions on where to get help.

How Stress Affects Your Health

It's no secret that stress can compromise your health. Continually tensed muscles cause pain, injury, headaches, backache, and eye muscle problems. A stressed heart and blood vessels can lead to clogged arteries, stroke, or heart attack. Stress increases acid production in the stomach and leads to heartburn and ulcers. Under stress, the immune system loses its ability to properly locate and fight infections. Even genetically programmed diseases can be triggered by the constant release of stress chemicals. Fibromyalgia is simply one in a long list of disorders directly related to stress.

Now that doctors understand the physiological mechanism responsible for fibromyalgia, we know that it is as biologically based as any other stress-related illness. Chronic stress resulting from emotional or physical pain causes fibromyalgia. The body does not discriminate between pain that stems from broken bones and pain that comes from a broken heart. In either case, the body's stress response goes into action, triggering a release of adrenaline, dopamine, and other fight-or-flight chemicals. In the short term, this rapid response serves you well, propelling you forward and hopefully beyond the initial crisis. Too often, however, the stress in your life is not readily alleviated, and the fight-or-flight response remains overactive, releasing a steady stream of stress hormones in an effort to keep you safely alert and on guard. Since you are already on edge, you are more easily aggravated, disturbed, irritable, and upset. With the fight-or-flight response on high alert, it becomes difficult to sleep, and even if you do sleep, it may not be the deep, restorative sleep you so desperately need. You can wind up trapped in a situation where the body is using up dopamine more quickly than it can be restored. Of course, with a diminished supply of dopamine, all your sensations become amplified, causing pain, discomfort, confusion, and even more stress.

The Anatomy of Stress

What is stress, anyway? Stress is the end result of your fight-or-flight response. The fight-or-flight response is only concerned with one thing: your survival. Think of stress hormones as human battery juice. Whenever this battery juice is released into your bloodstream, you are suddenly charged up to *do something* about the crisis at hand. In addition to your body's physiological reaction, an emotional reaction takes place. You may feel angry, sad, frustrated, or anxious. Emotions are an integral part of the fight-or-flight response. Generated on an unconscious level in the more primitive part of the brain, powerful emotions encourage you to move, to take action, to do something about a threat. Emotions have great power over you precisely because they are intended to save your life. If they didn't, you would be less likely to do something about a threat to your survival.

If you find yourself trapped in a fire, the powerful combination of physiological and emotional changes called stress could make the difference between life and death. However, when someone cuts you off in traffic, this same flood of chemicals does far more harm than good. There is nothing you can do about the traffic, and although it may be frustrating, it's certainly not life-threatening. Unfortunately, in today's fast-paced world, the fight-or-flight response engages easily throughout the day, triggering a cascade of hormones and evoking intense emotions. Far from helping you solve daily dilemmas, an unchecked fight-or-flight response puts you on an emotional roller coaster. You are continually thrown into a state of arousal in situations that are far from life-threatening.

It's not just you; it's everyone. It's a modern plague. If you have any doubts about being stuck in your own fight-or-flight response, consider the following questions:

- Do you feel stressed?
- Are you too preoccupied with the details of your own and other people's lives?
- Do you feel restless at night and have a hard time shutting off your mind?
- Can you relax only after you finish all the items on your to-do list?
- Does it seem impossible to simply sit in a chair and do nothing?

If you answered yes to two or more of these questions, it is likely that you are suffering from chronic stress. Once you have fibromyalgia, stress is your biggest enemy. Any additional activation of the fight-or-flight response is an obstacle to your recovery and is sure to lead to more pain. An argument with your child, frustration at being stuck in traffic, or depression about your illness—any of these will trigger your fight-or-flight response and get in the way of breaking the fibromyalgia cycle. In my attempts to counsel patients, I've learned that it doesn't do much good to recommend that people be less stressed and get good sleep. If you're like most of my patients, you would just tell me that most of the stress in your life is unavoidable. Your job is stressful, but you have to work to pay your bills. Your kids and family create a lot of stress, but you love them, and they're not going anywhere. You're already too busy, and now I want you to find the time to exercise and go to the grocery store instead of driving through at a fast-food restaurant. Even that seemingly small decision can impact your stress levels if you let it.

The fight-or-flight response runs on autopilot. Automatic reactions to life-threatening situations keep individuals alive. But when you have fibromyalgia, your automatic response system is on overdrive. The solution is to make the switch from autopilot to manual and take charge of your body's response to stress. You can't control stressful situations, but you can control your body's response to them. You've been taken on a wild ride for a long time, and now, you belong in the driver's seat. Get ready for your first lesson.

When you're an infant, your mind is essentially a blank slate. Your basic instincts motivate you to eat, drink, and seek warmth. Your brain's sole function is to ensure your survival. This is the job of your primitive mind. You don't have a lot of unnecessary fears or concerns. Over time, you learn fear as your basic needs are incompletely met and you feel discomfort. A variety of life experiences program different fears into your mind. Consider how fears and attachments develop very early in life. A warm and dry newborn with a full belly is satisfied and content. In the beginning, a baby can be picked up by anyone without crying. However, a baby soon learns that his mother is more likely to keep him safe and meet his needs than anyone else. He begins to associate a sense of security with the mother and will feel safer with her than with anyone else. Now, if the baby is hungry and someone else picks him up, he is more likely to cry in frustration or fear. This is the beginning of a lifelong process that shapes the way the fight-or-flight response is triggered so that it more specifically meets situational environmental challenges. This is something that all species do throughout their lifetimes. Inevitably, as the child grows, his fight-or-flight response will develop a long set of learned triggers.

We are born into an uncertain world. As a result, the fight-or-flight response is continually reassessing the outside world for threats in order to try to maintain a sense of security.

As the thinking brain, or higher mind, engages, an entirely new set of fears emerges—What do people think of me? Am I pretty enough? Why can't I drive a nicer car? None of us enter the world worried about whether our baby blanket matches our booties. As a baby, you're content just to be warm. In general, most of the things that make us feel threatened are learned responses. If you could take your checkbook back in time to a cave man and explain how you have plenty to eat but your dwindling bank balance is causing high blood pressure, you wouldn't get much sympathy. Unfortunately, it is this constant redefining of how the fight-or-flight response is used that leads to most of the stress in our lives.

Reprogramming the Fight-or-Flight Response

The adrenaline release caused by stressful thoughts and the subsequent cascade of emotions feels so uncontrollable precisely because it is uncontrollable—at first. Although the initial activation of the fight-or-flight response happens automatically, you can learn to stop the process before it goes too far. Once the fight-or-flight response starts, you can choose how to respond to the anger, frustration, or anxiety it generates.

Most people are relying on an exhaustive security list that was generated unconsciously. For you to modify this list and gain control over your own brain, you first have to identify when you are initiating (and trapping yourself in) the fight-or-flight response. Over time, you can eliminate most unnecessary fight-or-flight triggers. All of my patients who succeed in controlling their fight-or-flight response do so by learning the triad. The triad is a sequence of three steps that effectively shuts off the autopilot and puts you in control:

Step 1: Recognize the Fight-or-Flight Feeling
Step 2: Identify the Misguided Security Need
Step 3: Do the Opposite

Step 1: Recognize the Fight-or-Flight Feeling

Start paying attention to the daily fluctuation in emotions you experience. What if you finish grocery shopping and realize you can't find your wallet when it's time to check out? It's not in your purse, and you can't remember where it is. The clerk has already scanned your groceries, and there is a long line of people behind you. How do you feel? Ask yourself the following questions:

- Is my fight-or-flight response active?
- Do I feel any of the negative emotions associated with the fight-or-flight response?

You may feel anxiety, fear, anger, or even stress. However, these sensations and emotions can be subtle, depending on the situation. You should also pay attention to:

- judgments
- feelings of injustice
- blaming others
- blaming yourself; beating yourself up inside
- attachment to others' words and actions
- fear of rejection or acceptance
- envy
- doing too much to please or help others

The negative emotions generated by the primitive mind are the key to knowing when your fight-or-flight response is active.

Whenever you feel stress, anger, anxiety, or frustration, there is no question that you are being motivated by the primitive mind in its single-minded genetic goal to ensure your survival. Does a misplaced wallet actually merit this flood of emotion? The primitive mind is operating off a misguided security need—your survival is not actually threatened!

Step 2: Identify the Misguided Security Need

Every time you look outside yourself for security, your fight-or-flight response starts acting up. By looking outside, I mean getting your security needs met through the actions of others. This also includes everything that happens outside you, including the weather, the stock market, the condition of your car or house, and even the way your partner puts the toilet paper on the holder. Whenever you identify the fight-or-flight feeling, ask yourself the following questions:

- Is this situation threatening my life, my family, or my safety?
- What will happen if I can't meet this need?
- Is this situation worth using up my adrenaline and going into emotional high gear?
- Is there any advantage in not letting this go in order to let myself feel better?
- Is it worth a fibromyalgia flare?

Does losing your wallet constitute a threat to your food, shelter, or safety? No. The fight-or-flight response doesn't see it that way. What's your misguided security threat? You may be worried about being late or making a fool of yourself in the checkout line. You may even go into panic mode over what might have happened to your wallet. Although these may constitute legitimate concerns, each one actually represents a misguided security need.

Make sure you pay attention when the security need is appropriate. If you are being physically threatened, I encourage you to get your adrenaline up and do something about it. Fight back or run away. However, if the need is for anything other than your ability to protect yourself or your family, it is an inappropriate security need.

Step 3: Do the Opposite

The main goal in step 3 is to avoid doing what the fight-or-flight response is telling you to do. You'll come to find that if you don't follow the directives of the fight-or-flight response and nothing bad happens, your brain will eventually learn to stop overreacting. When you do this, your brain experiences the opposite of what you fear and learns that your survival is not at stake. This is the only way to stop the involuntary fight-or-flight response that is currently controlling your thoughts and actions.

Let's go back to the lost wallet example. It's amazing how something as simple as misplacing your wallet can quickly trigger fight-or-flight emotions. You feel embarrassed because you're at the front of a long checkout line, and now you are holding it up. You may feel the urge to yell at your children, blame your husband, or even act like it's the cashier's fault. None of these reactions will solve the problem—they'll simply send your adrenaline levels skyrocketing. Do the opposite. Recognize that your emotions stem from a misguided security need—the desire to look competent in front of other people. Tell yourself that nothing about the current situation actually merits a fight-or-flight reaction. Shut down the fight-or-flight response by taking a deep breath and calmly explaining the situation to the cashier. Don't yell at your kids or blame your husband—that simply fuels the fight-or-flight response. Once your groceries have been set aside, you can look for your wallet, call a friend, or do something constructive to remedy the situation. The next time you encounter a similar situation, your brain may not be as quick to identify it as a security threat.

Another way to diffuse the fight-or-flight response is to share your fears with someone you trust. Any problem that is shared with another human being loses its grip on you. The worst thing you can ever do about an inappropriate fight-or-flight response is act out on what the primitive mind is telling you to do. Furthermore, you absolutely must not stew, or stay alone in your head (in the primitive mind), over the problem. Unfortunately, you will receive overwhelming urges to do just that. It can be frightening to share your personal fears with anyone else. When you are in self-protection mode, the thought of exposing yourself to even your best friend can seem like too big a risk. However, once you share your fears with someone else, they will lose some of their power over you.

As I travel from city to city, speaking about fibromyalgia and the fight-or-flight response, many people generously share with me the details of their personal lives and tell me about their problems. As I listen, there seems to be one common theme: no matter how simple or complicated a problem, the fight-or-flight response is always so overwhelming for them that the primitive mind's message becomes irresistible. I teach them how to resist this message and apply my triad instead. It is the key to their freedom from stress. When you change a negative thought, you will always change the subsequent emotional feelings that are sent to your body. If this seems hard to believe, think back to when you had a good week with your fibromyalgia. You probably had less stress, and you slept better. The reason for this good week was that you spent less time experiencing the fight-or-flight response.

Apply the triad to little things. Don't tackle the thirty-year-old fight with your mother-in-law just yet; start with how you feel when you hear the alarm clock ring. First, identify when you are in fight-or-flight mode by observing your emotions. Then, begin to apply the triad. Go slowly. It can take a long time to undo destructive thinking habits, but it is well worth it.

To get a sense of just how active your fight-or-flight response is, record in your Progress Journal for several days anything that triggers a surge of adrenaline. Be sure to pay attention to the small stressors as well as the more obvious ones. Review these stressors and practice applying the triad to each of them. After you have been using the triad for two weeks, take a day to once again record anything that triggers your fight-or-flight response. If you repeat this exercise every few weeks, you'll not only be able to track your progress but you'll also become more aware of which fight-or-flight triggers need the most work.

Establish Proper Boundaries

After you have been practicing the triad for a while, it becomes almost automatic to shut down your fight-or-flight response over misguided security needs. Getting cut off in traffic, being late for an appointment, or coming home to a messy house will no longer trigger a flood of adrenaline. Controlling your fight-or-flight response in the context of a relationship is another matter entirely. We actually do *need* other people. Humans are a social species, and our brains are genetically programmed to establish and maintain relationships. No matter how difficult other people make your life, your brain instinctively places tremendous importance on maintaining these connections. You need far more than the mere physical presence of other people—you need love, understanding, and support. This isn't just a feel-good message. These things help ensure your very survival. When human babies are raised in sterile, emotionless environments, they die in a matter of weeks or months, no matter how well their other basic needs are met. The odds of surviving a heart attack, cancer, or stroke increase for people with a strong social network. It's also no coincidence that people who live with other people live longer than those who live alone. You need other people, and your brain knows it. We all think that people stay in bad relationships because of their hearts, but actually, it's all in their heads. Navigating the emotional ups and downs of a relationship is challenging, because other people actually represent an important security need in your life. If you have an argument or misunderstanding with someone you love, your brain may perceive it as a threat to your welfare. As a result, the people you care about the most are the most likely to trigger your fight-or-flight response.

Fortunately, there are things you can do to control this. First, work on controlling your fight-or-flight response around other people. Practice this with everyone you encounter. It's generally easier with people you don't know as well. When someone you don't care about rubs you the wrong way, it only takes a little practice to identify your misguided security need and move on. The more intimate the relationship, the more challenging it is to control your fight-or-flight response. The fight-or-flight response expresses itself in many different ways. If you have a secure relationship with someone, you may be more likely to reveal your fight-or-flight feelings because you know they won't leave. However, if you have a shaky relationship with someone you care about, your fight-or-flight response might engage precisely because you're afraid he or she will leave.

With a lot of practice, you will become better and better at keeping your cool with other people. But what if you control your own fight-or-flight response, but your spouse, parent, or friend doesn't control his or hers? What if this person just keeps coming at you with his or her own fight-or-flight response? You may find yourself engaging in stupid arguments even when you know it isn't worthwhile.

Developing healthy interpersonal boundaries is the key to keeping your fight-or-flight response in check in the most difficult of situations. Proper boundaries prevent a conversation with someone else from turning into a fight-or-flight trigger for you. In order to maintain proper boundaries with other people, you will have to become consciously assertive toward others about your needs. If you feel a conversation is going downhill and you are starting to feel defensive, upset, or angry, it's time for you to redirect the conversation. Establishing a proper boundary might consist of a request to continue a conversation later: "I can tell that we are both starting to get upset. Why don't we continue this conversation when we've had a chance to calm down." Another tactic might be to set ground rules for the conversation: "I'd like to continue this conversation, but we are both getting upset. Can we both agree not to interrupt or raise our voices at one another?" As you become better at controlling your fight-or-flight response, you'll also become more comfortable with knowing when to establish a boundary. You will always know when you have not protected or haven't even created your boundaries, because your fight-or-flight response will go into action.

Practice Constructive Communication

In my research into human stress and chronic pain, I learned a great way to express my needs without threatening others from Dr. Marshall Rosenberg's book *Nonviolent Communication*. This is an excellent reference for people who want to improve their communication skills and develop more intimate relationships with other individuals. Dr. Rosenberg describes four basic steps to successful communication:

1. First, reflect back what the other person has said or done. Express what you observe without blame, criticism, or judgment. If someone made you angry by leaving the room and slamming the door in anger, you would observe "When you left the room…" rather than "I can't believe you left the room like that!"
2. Express the feeling in you that is affected by the person's words or actions. You are letting the person know that what he or she says or does affects the way you feel. Be sure to stick with feelings and avoid judgments. "When you left the room, I felt sad" expresses emotion. A person can relate to this without feeling blamed or getting defensive. If you say, "When you left the room, I felt ignored," you are conveying judgment. The other person may hear "You ignored me" and get defensive. *Angry, sad, glad,* and *afraid* are all words that express the root feeling and avoid judgment.
3. Validate your own needs by stating them. State the need you would like this person to meet: "I need more respect."
4. Make a specific request, but don't make a demand: "In the future, I'd appreciate it if you would ask for a break in the conversation before leaving the room."

Following Dr. Rosenberg's technique means letting go of being right and creating a space in which two people can hear each other without judgment and blame. I always add a fifth step to this process. In addition to Rosenberg's four steps, try to say something reassuring right after you state your need and before you make your request. This will help indicate that you hear, understand, and care about the other person. It might sound like this: "I need more respect. *I understand that you left the room because you were really angry and didn't know how else to show your anger.* In the future..."

Let's look at an example. Barbara feels frustrated because every day after work, her husband, John, turns the television on and tunes her out. In the past, whenever she has tried to talk to him about her concerns, their conversations have quickly disintegrated into angry accusations that left her feeling even more distraught. She knows she can't continue to ignore the problem, because every evening, her fight-or-flight response kicks in as soon as John flips on the TV. Her fight-or-flight response urges her to be angry and defensive when she talks to John about the problem. However, if Barbara uses the model described above, she is much more likely to have a nonthreatening and constructive conversation with her husband. She will also be doing the opposite of what her fight-or-flight response is telling her to do, which is the final step of the triad.

She might say something like the following:

> When you come home from work and watch television for the rest of the evening, I feel lonely. I want to feel connected to you. I know that when you come home from work, you're tired and want to zone out. I would appreciate it if we could find time each evening to check in with each other. I want to hear about your day and tell you about my day. It would be great if we could go for a walk, have dinner together, or just talk for a few minutes before you start watching television.

There is nothing threatening about this approach. Barbara doesn't blame her husband or demand that he change his routine. She tells him how his actions make her feel without putting him down or judging him for his actions. She gives him every chance of seeing her need and responding to her request in an equally nonconfrontational way.

For someone stuck in fight-or-flight mode, the above example might seem scary or even impossible. The primitive mind doesn't want the battle to end; it wants to win. In order to truly deactivate your fight-or-flight response around other people, you're going to have to throw right and wrong out the window. The goal is no longer to win the argument but to replace a battle of wills with a constructive conversation. Using effective communication techniques with proper boundaries in place is the best way to approach another person who is stuck in fight-or-flight mode. Remember:

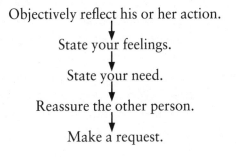

Objectively reflect his or her action.

State your feelings.

State your need.

Reassure the other person.

Make a request.

Asking for Help

If you follow the suggestions above, you'll make headway against the seemingly pervasive stress of daily life. For some people, this advice is all they really need to make some big changes in their lives. However, I encourage my patients to look to outside sources for help as well. Battling fibromyalgia is difficult, and you should enlist all the support you can find. Many counselors and therapists are trained to help people work through such difficult illnesses as fibromyalgia. A good cognitive-behavioral therapist or counselor will understand how to help you work through the psychological triggers of the fight-or-flight response. The therapist will not only provide you with emotional support but can help keep you on track as you work toward making difficult changes in your life.

If you find that the biggest source of stress in your life comes from your spouse, a parent, or a child, consider going to marriage or family counseling with that person. Resolving challenging emotional issues is a tremendous step in the direction of recovery. If you've never been to a counselor or therapist, ask your doctor to recommend one. Also, keep in mind that every counselor is different, and you might have to interview a few before you find one who really works for you.

All by itself, the stress of having fibromyalgia is reason enough to find a good counselor. There are several other situations that also merit getting professional help. For some people, depression is a key fibromyalgia trigger. Other people develop signs of clinical depression after they have suffered from fibromyalgia. While major depression occurs in almost 10 percent of adults, it is present in approximately 30 percent of fibromyalgia patients. If you suffer from depression, you may find it extremely difficult to find the motivation you need to get well. People with depression cannot just "pull themselves together." It is a clinical disorder, and as an illness, it is every bit as real as fibromyalgia. If you suffer from depression, it is important to ask for help. Depression is treatable, and your doctor can help you decide the best approach to take.

You should also seek professional help for other types of psychological disorders, such as bipolar disorder or posttraumatic stress disorder. These are challenging conditions, and without treatment, they are likely to keep you trapped in the fibromyalgia cycle indefinitely. Fortunately, these conditions are more thoroughly understood now than they were in the past, and help is available.

I also recommend finding a fibromyalgia support group. Although your family and friends may be supportive, they will never understand what it is like to have fibromyalgia. You can alleviate a lot of stress by connecting with other people who truly understand what you are going through. You can find a partial listing of fibromyalgia support groups by state at www.fmaware.org. Unless you live in a big city, you may have trouble finding a fibromyalgia support group. Even if you do find one, its meetings may not fit into your schedule. For that reason, I created The Forum. The Forum is an online discussion group that puts people with fibromyalgia in touch with one another. You will have the opportunity to share your experiences and meet others who are facing similar challenges. The Forum has a section devoted to the fight-or-flight response. Just like this book, The Forum is for people focused on curing fibromyalgia, not just learning to live with it. You can sign up for The Forum on my Web site: www.drdryland.com.

Other Ways to Alleviate Stress

Applying the triad to stressful situations is the most effective way to control your fight-or-flight response. However, this won't happen overnight. It will take time, practice, and possibly the help of a good counselor or therapist. In the meantime, there are some other things you can do on a daily or weekly basis to help alleviate the harmful effects of stress on your body. The following is a list of helpful stress reducers.

Meditation

Western science is finally starting to show clear-cut evidence that meditation plays an important role in reducing the harmful effects of stress. Meditation counters the effects of the sympathetic nervous system, the branch of the autonomic nervous system responsible for the fight-or-flight response. A daily meditative practice basically trains your brain to relax, effectively resetting the sensitivity of your fight-or-flight trigger. Multiple studies have found that meditation reduces the levels of hormones associated with stress and improves health. Because meditation effectively counters the effects of stress, it improves sleep and bolsters the immune system. In one remarkable study, researchers found that people who practiced meditation for four months produced more antibodies to a flu shot than did people who didn't practice meditation. An increase in antibodies signified an important increase in their overall immune response. In another study, fibromyalgia patients participated in a ten-week meditation program. Everyone who completed the program showed improvement in one or more of the following categories: global well-being, pain, sleep, or fatigue.

So what is meditation, exactly, and how can you do it? Meditation is a conscious effort to relax your mind. When you meditate, you learn to let go of attachment to the thoughts that enter and leave your mind. Normally, when a thought enters your mind, you either let it go or grab on to it and start analyzing. Meditating involves letting go of thoughts rather than holding on tight. To check out meditation for yourself, do the following:

1. Find a quiet place where you can sit comfortably for five to twenty minutes. Try to sit with your back straight, rather than slouching or leaning. However, if you need support, you can sit with your back against a wall or in a chair. Set a timer if it will help keep you from worrying about how long you have been meditating.

2. Close your eyes, and consciously let go of any tension you are holding in your body. Relax your shoulders, unclench your fists, and soften your face.

3. Slowly become aware of your breathing. Concentrate on the air coming in through your nose, filling your lungs, and then once again leaving your body. Breathe in a slow and natural rhythm. You can continue to concentrate only on your breath, in and out, or you can choose a word or short phrase to focus on.

4. As you concentrate on your breathing or word, be aware that thoughts will naturally come into your mind. Observe your thoughts and emotions without attachment, and let them go. Return to your breathing. Do not be frustrated by distracting thoughts. Do not judge yourself on your ability to clear your mind. Continue to use your breathing as an anchor, returning to it over and over again.

5. When the timer goes off or you are ready to quit, open your eyes and sit quietly for another minute or two before getting up.

There is nothing complicated about setting up a daily meditation practice. If you are at all intrigued, I highly recommend that you give it a try. There are many books and resources on meditation, some of which are listed in the resources section at the end of this book. You can learn about different techniques online or even find classes on meditation.

Breathing Exercises

Controlling your breathing can be a powerful way to control your emotions as well. Meditation, yoga, Pilates, tai chi, and many other practices use breathing as a grounding and stabilizing force.

When you are not conscious of your breathing, this mirrors your state of mind. People who have panic attacks may hyperventilate, while people who are deeply relaxed take slow, easy breaths. It can work the other way around as well. When you feel your emotions rising, pay attention to your breathing. Slowly and consciously inhale and exhale, letting the rhythm of your breathing slow your heart rate and calm your mind. Once you have slowed your emotional response, apply the triad.

Find Gratitude

When you have fibromyalgia, it's easy and even natural to focus on the problems in your life. It becomes habit to focus on the bad things that have happened to you and to forget about the positive. These negative thought patterns will only increase your stress level and make the fibromyalgia cycle worse. Try something totally different for a change. At the end of each day, write down all the things you are grateful for in your Progress Journal. If you can't think of much, go back to the basics. Be grateful that you are safe and have food to eat and a warm place to sleep. Be grateful that you care enough to read this book and haven't totally given up. Find gratitude in friends, a blue sky, or even a funny TV show. Stretch your imagination, and go out of your way to find things to be grateful for. This simple task can help train your brain to once again focus on the positive.

Exercise

Daily exercise is a proven stress reducer. Exercise responds to the fight-or-flight response's insistent call to action, causing the stress hormones in your system to dissipate. However, most people with fibromyalgia find exercise difficult because of pain and fatigue. Chapter 9 explains how you can successfully find an exercise program that works for your body.

Release Through Writing

Another way to let go of stressful or upsetting thoughts is to write them down. Sometimes, you have to literally say something or write it down in order to let go of it. If you are inclined to write, devote some time each day to writing down your thoughts and feelings. If you can get something down on paper, it will oftentimes lose any power it formerly had over you. Journaling will also help you better understand your fight-or-flight triggers, as they are sure to surface whenever you write down your thoughts.

In a Nutshell . . .

- Stress and physical pain are often so interconnected that you can't resolve one without resolving the other.
- In today's stressful world, the fight-or-flight response is overactive. You must learn to consciously control your fight-or-flight response. Over time, you can reprogram your brain from a state of stress to a state of calm.
- Use the triad to manually control your fight-or-flight response: (1) recognize the fight-or-flight feeling, (2) identify the misguided security need, and (3) do the opposite of your instinctual reaction.
- Controlling your fight-or-flight response is very difficult in close relationships. Learn how to establish proper boundaries with other people and improve your communication skills.
- Other effective techniques for controlling your fight-or-flight response include meditation, breathing exercises, finding gratitude, exercise, and journaling.
- Controlling your fight-or-flight response will not only improve your fibromyalgia symptoms, it will improve your entire life.

CHAPTER 8

Eating Well and Feeling Better

The last two chapters went right to the root causes of fibromyalgia and explained how resolving issues related to sleep and stress can jump-start your recovery. This chapter focuses on something almost as important: your diet. When I lead seminars on fibromyalgia, I am inevitably asked about the relationship between food and fibromyalgia. Do some foods make fibromyalgia worse? Is there a fibromyalgia diet? What can I eat to feel better? Some people with fibromyalgia intuitively sense that there is some kind of relationship between the food they eat and how they feel. They're exactly right. This may seem odd, because you're probably eating the same foods you've been eating your entire life. Why are you having problems with them now? Although diet does not cause fibromyalgia, once your sensations are amplified, your diet can become one of the biggest contributors to your symptoms.

There are a variety of ways in which the food you eat can have a dramatic impact on the way you feel on a daily basis. If you have fibromyalgia, there's a good chance you suffer from food-related headaches, irritable bowel syndrome, food allergies or food intolerances, hypoglycemia, or other problems related to the regulation of blood glucose levels. In addition, different foods contribute to inflammation, fatigue, muscle pain, painful digestive problems, insomnia, and acid reflux—all of which are magnified by fibromyalgia. Poor eating habits can also weaken your immune system, leaving you even more susceptible to the common cold or a bad case of the flu. Even if you eat a relatively healthful diet, you are likely to have increased sensitivity to the negative effects of certain foods, creating an entirely different set of challenges for your body. As a consequence, controlling your diet is one of the most effective ways to control the way you feel each day.

There is no generic fibromyalgia diet. The dietary changes you need to make depend completely on your body and your symptoms. For some people, diet simply doesn't play a big role in exacerbating their symptoms. However, for others, making key dietary changes is one of the most effective, proven ways to reduce or eliminate many of their symptoms. Although changing your diet won't cure fibromyalgia, it can have a dramatic effect on your immune system, energy level, and general state of well-being. These changes can happen in a matter of weeks, giving you the extra energy you need to focus on other elements of your long-term recovery plan. Although you initially may need to make some big changes in your diet, these changes aren't forever. As you recover from fibromyalgia, you will once again be able to eat any of the foods you ate without problems before you developed fibromyalgia. In this chapter, you'll learn how to determine whether your current diet is making your symptoms worse and the important changes you can make to reduce your symptoms and start feeling better right away.

Your Diet Can Make Fibromyalgia Worse

There are two primary reasons that fibromyalgia patients have problems with certain kinds of food. The first of these is directly related to the fact that your sensation threshold is greatly reduced. Instead of being able to eat a large variety of foods with minimal or no side effects, you are now extremely sensitive to the ways in which your body reacts to foods. As a result, what used to be a mild bloating sensation after a heavy meal may now feel like unbearable pain and cramping in your abdomen. Different foods can contribute to aches and pains, headaches, fatigue, digestive problems, and even depression. Later in this chapter, you'll learn how to figure out which foods might be problem foods for you. The second problem with regard to food and fibromyalgia is that a prolonged activation of the fight-or-flight response can actually alter your body's ability to utilize, store, and release carbohydrates. I'll discuss this in more detail below. First, let's take a look at the different ways food can exacerbate your symptoms.

Foods That Cause Digestive Problems

Some foods are more difficult to digest than others, causing bloating, cramping, gas, diarrhea, and indigestion. Once you have fibromyalgia, these symptoms can become unbearable. Foods and beverages that are especially prone to causing digestive problems are dairy, corn, sugar, coffee, tea, eggs, beef, glutinous grains (wheat, barley, oats, rye, triticale, semolina, spelt, kamut, bulgur), and alcohol. Too much insoluble fiber (fiber that doesn't dissolve in water), which is found in grains and vegetables, can also cause digestive problems for some people.

Irritable Bowel Syndrome and Fibromyalgia

Irritable bowel syndrome (IBS) is a common problem associated with the lower digestive tract. The symptoms of IBS include abdominal pain, heartburn, constipation, and diarrhea. Fibromyalgia and IBS have remarkably similar triggers, including stress, poor sleep, posttraumatic stress disorder, depression, and anxiety. Consequently, there is almost a 70 percent overlap between the two conditions. IBS can make anyone miserable, and that's even more true for a fibromyalgia patient. If you have IBS, it is especially important to avoid or greatly reduce your intake of foods that could trigger an episode of IBS. Many of these are the same foods that cause the digestive problems listed above. The consumption of fatty foods is problematic for people with IBS, as the fat triggers the colon to start contracting, resulting in pain and discomfort. Other trigger foods include red meat, dark poultry meat, dairy products, egg yolks, and fried foods. Foods that cause gas, acidic foods, and foods high in fructose are also problematic. Too much insoluble fiber is also a problem for people with IBS, although a certain amount of roughage is necessary for any healthful diet. With IBS, as with anything else, the trick lies in identifying your problem foods and learning how to either reduce or eliminate these from your diet.

Gluten Intolerance

Intolerance to gluten is one of the most common and overlooked food sensitivities. Gluten is the elastic protein that makes bread dough sticky. It is found in grains from the wheat family, which includes barley, oats, and rye. With fibromyalgia, a previously undetectable gluten intolerance could cause many of your symptoms. In addition to such physical symptoms as gas, bloating, diarrhea, and abdominal pain, gluten intolerance is linked to irritability, depression, muscle cramps, joint pain, and fatigue. A negative reaction to gluten may occur over the course of days, weeks, or even months. The elimination/ challenge diet described below will give you an opportunity to see whether eliminating gluten will help reduce your symptoms.

Lactose Intolerance

Another common food problem is an intolerance to lactose, a type of sugar found in milk products. The symptoms of lactose intolerance generally occur within a few hours of consuming lactose. They are generally gastrointestinal and include nausea, abdominal cramps and bloating, gas, and diarrhea but can also include fatigue and headache. As with gluten, you may be more aware of difficulties with lactose now that you have fibromyalgia.

Inflammatory Foods

Some foods cause an inflammatory response that can lead to mild to pronounced swelling in the muscles, joints, and other parts of the body. If you suffer from underlying medical or physical conditions made worse by inflammation, such as rheumatoid arthritis or tendonitis, any added inflammation will cause pain and contribute to your discomfort. Foods that are especially high in sugar and saturated fat, which includes junk food, highly processed foods, and fast food, have been linked to inflammation. Red meat, eggs, and wheat contain an acid that, when consumed in large amounts, contributes to inflammation. Vegetables in the nightshade family, including tomatoes, eggplant, and potatoes, can also make inflammation worse. Alcohol and caffeine also exacerbate inflammation.

Excitotoxins: MSG and Aspartame

Monosodium glutamate (MSG) and aspartame are both excitotoxins. Excitotoxins are molecules that have been shown to cause neurological damage. One small study found that the elimination of MSG and aspartame from the diet alleviated most fibromyalgia symptoms for a very limited number of patients. These are both food additives that act as excitatory neurotransmitters and may exacerbate fibromyalgia symptoms. MSG enhances the flavor of foods and is frequently used in Asian restaurants; you can usually ask for dishes made without MSG. Aspartame, also known as NutraSweet, is a sweetener commonly used in diet soft drinks and other foods. One of the byproducts of aspartame is formaldehyde—the same thing as embalming fluid. Instead of helping you lose weight, aspartame actually *protects your fat cells from being broken down*. Do yourself a favor and avoid MSG and aspartame.

Foods Linked to Headaches

Most people with fibromyalgia suffer more than their share of headaches. Headaches are triggered by a variety of changes in the body, and when you have fibromyalgia, you are sensitive to even a mild change in sinus pressure or other headache triggers. For some people, certain foods are more likely than others to trigger headaches. Coffee, tea, and chocolate, all of which contain caffeine, can trigger headaches either through consumption or withdrawal. Such food additives and preservatives as

MSG, nitrites, and nitrates trigger headaches for some people. Aged cheeses and cultured dairy products are also a cause of headaches. Everyone is different, and what triggers a headache for one person might be fine for another. I recommend paying close attention to whether certain foods seem to cause headaches. Later in this chapter, I'll explain how keeping a food journal can help you identify problem foods, such as headache triggers. As I'll discuss below, you may also be more susceptible to blood sugar swings, increasing the number of headaches you experience.

Problems with Carbohydrate Utilization, Storage, and Release

People with fibromyalgia often have problems with the utilization, storage, and release of carbohydrates. Unlike the other food problems we've discussed that are directly related to the hypersensitivity that characterizes fibromyalgia, this problem is more directly related to a prolonged activation of the fight-or-flight response. Chronic activation of the fight-or-flight response interferes with the process that stabilizes blood sugar levels as carbohydrates are digested. Adrenaline plays an important role in the digestive process, ensuring that your body has enough glucose (blood sugar) available for quick energy, should it be needed. However, when your fight-or-flight response has been overactive for a long time, your adrenaline levels, while not as depleted as dopamine, are stretched thin, interfering with the process that keeps your blood glucose levels stable.

As an example, many people with fibromyalgia suffer from reactive hypoglycemia. Rather than maintaining a constant level of available glucose, the body overreacts to the consumption of simple carbohydrates (carbohydrates that break down rapidly into sugar) by releasing too much insulin. Insulin facilitates the conversion of glucose to body fat and causes a rapid drop in blood sugar. When your blood sugar drops rapidly, the body perceives a threat, and the fight-or-flight response goes into action. A shot of adrenaline assists in activating the release of sugars stored as glycogen in the liver and muscles. The symptoms of reactive hypoglycemia—sweating, weakness, hunger, anxiety, numbness, and tingling—result from the release of adrenaline into the bloodstream. However, when you have fibromyalgia, your overworked sympathetic nervous system may not have enough adrenaline in reserve to stabilize blood glucose levels. As a result, you may continue to crave simple carbohydrates and sugars in a futile attempt to bring your blood glucose level back into balance. Later in this chapter, I'll discuss how you can counter this problem by making some basic dietary adjustments.

Common Fibromyalgia Problem Foods

There are some foods (and drinks) you should either consume in moderation or stay away from altogether while you have fibromyalgia because they are most likely to exacerbate or even cause some of your symptoms. If you stay away from these items, it's likely that many of your symptoms will subside, and you'll find that you lose your craving for these items altogether:

Refined Sugar

When you eat refined sugar (like table sugar, high-fructose corn syrup, corn syrup, and sucrose), your metabolism bursts into a roaring glucose-fueled blaze that suddenly goes out, creating the hypoglycemic state. Your body then releases adrenaline in an attempt to stabilize blood glucose levels, taxing your already overworked adrenal glands. In addition, consuming too much sugar depresses your immune system and is linked to chronic inflammation and many other health problems. It is easy to dramatically decrease your intake of refined sugars simply by reading food labels and paying more attention to what you eat. You should definitely eliminate sugar-loaded soft drinks, candy, and other sweets. Try products made with stevia. They contain the leaf of a tropical herb that is many hundreds of times sweeter than table sugar and does not cause your blood sugar to spike. Since it is so sweet, you should use far less than you would with other sweeteners.

Caffeine

Caffeine is a stimulant, meaning that it triggers the same stress hormones used by the fight-or-flight response to give you a short-lived burst of energy. Caffeine only serves to exacerbate the problems caused by an overactive fight-or-flight response. If you think caffeine doesn't affect you, it's probably because your adrenaline is too depleted to respond appropriately. Caffeine causes acid reflux, inhibits the absorption of some nutrients, irritates the urinary tract and bladder, increases the risk of osteoarthritis, impairs concentration over time, and causes significant blood sugar swings. Caffeine is linked to almost every symptom fibromyalgia patients experience, including irritability, anxiety, headaches, and interrupted sleep. Caffeine is also a diuretic, causing most people who drink it to be chronically dehydrated. To avoid headaches and other symptoms of withdrawal, reduce your caffeine use gradually. Substitute green or black teas in the beginning. Most people who stop using caffeine are surprised to find that their energy levels climb and stay consistently higher. If you can't give up caffeine entirely, green tea is the best option. Limit your intake to one to two cups a day.

Red Meat

Red meat contributes to inflammation, causes digestive problems, triggers IBS, contains high levels of saturated fats, and causes many other health problems over the long term. It's easy to substitute fish or poultry for red meat.

Alcohol

In recent years, there has been a lot of press about the benefits of moderate alcohol use. Limited consumption is linked to increased heart health and may help protect you from type 2 diabetes and gallstones. However, if you have fibromyalgia, alcohol most likely does more harm than good. Alcohol disrupts sleep—one of your most important allies in the fight against fibromyalgia. Alcohol also contributes to blood sugar swings and may have negative interactions with some of the medications you are currently taking. Until your fibromyalgia is under control, I recommend eliminating or greatly moderating alcohol consumption. At most, you should limit yourself to one or two glasses of red wine a week.

What Does the Research Say?

There haven't been a lot of big studies on diet and fibromyalgia, but two small studies have yielded some rather remarkable results. Each study observed significant improvements in fibromyalgia patients who followed strict vegetarian diets. In a year 2000 controlled study at the University of Kuopio in Finland, eighteen fibromyalgia patients followed a low-salt, strictly vegan (no animal products), raw food diet for three months. Their results were compared to those of fifteen women with fibromyalgia who continued their normal diets. At the end of three months, participants who followed the vegan diet had significant improvements in pain, joint stiffness, quality of sleep, and morning stiffness.

In 2001, thirty people in North Carolina participated in a study in which they ate a mostly raw, purely vegetarian diet for up to seven months. Twenty people followed the diet through to the completion of the study. Over half of the participants showed significant improvement in their physical functioning, general health, vitality, social functioning, and emotional and mental health at the end of two months. These participants did not see a significant improvement in overall body pain but did improve on other pain scores. More improvements were seen at the end of four months, and the results remained stable at the end of seven months. At the conclusion of the study, the general health, vitality, and emotional and mental health scores of those participants classified as responders (nineteen participants) improved to *normal* levels after nothing more than some rather strict dietary changes.

Why did most of the people who participated in these studies see some rather dramatic improvements in their symptoms? My suspicion is that by following a mostly raw, vegetarian diet, they automatically eliminated most of the problem foods described above. They weren't necessarily resolving the root cause of fibromyalgia, but they were successfully reducing triggers. These studies demonstrate the important role dietary changes can play in helping you down the path to recovery. How do I know that they weren't actually curing fibromyalgia? Well, following a vegetarian and especially a vegan diet is extremely challenging, and few people have the discipline to stick it out. In fact, none of the participants in the vegan diet study continued the diet after the initial three months. Their symptoms returned once they reverted to eating their previous diets because they still had fibromyalgia. Another reason study participants probably felt better is that they were eating a lot of fresh, raw foods. Raw foods contain enzymes that assist with digestion and also contain higher levels of nutrients than do cooked or processed foods. Raw foods are also full of immune-boosting antioxidants.

You can make similar dietary changes to start feeling better now. According to these studies, the biggest results are evident in as little as two months and plateau at four months. I've had patients who felt tremendously better within weeks of switching to a strictly controlled diet. The good news is that you won't have to stay on a strict diet forever. Once you recover, your fibromyalgia-induced food problems will disappear, as you will no longer be hypersensitive to the effects of different foods. Fortunately, even now, you don't need to follow the exceedingly strict diets used in these studies to achieve significant improvements in your own physical and mental health.

The Three-Week Elimination/Challenge Diet

As we discussed above, it is extremely likely that some component of your diet greatly contributes to your symptoms. If you can identify problem foods and eliminate them, you will have taken an important step toward recovery. Food doesn't cause fibromyalgia, and diet changes alone won't cure fibromyalgia. However, becoming aware of and eliminating problem foods can help you feel better than you have in weeks, months, or even years and give you the strength to take on the true causes of fibromyalgia. I recommend a three-week protocol that eliminates all the fibromyalgia problem foods described earlier in this chapter. If you have other health-related dietary needs, talk to your doctor before following this protocol.

This is not really a diet. It is a diagnostic tool to discover whether you have problem foods or sensitivities you may have been previously unaware of. During the first three weeks, you will eliminate potentially problematic foods. After this initial period, you will then challenge your body by reintroducing each food. Three weeks is not a very long time to follow this protocol, especially when you consider how long you have already been sick. Compared to the suffering you have endured, following a three-week diet with the potential to give you tremendous health benefits is about as close to instant gratification as fibromyalgia patients can get. People generally have trouble sticking to diets because they know if they cheat, they can always start over tomorrow. This protocol is different. Once you start, you can't cheat, unless you want to start the three weeks completely over. This protocol isn't about losing weight, it's about feeling better.

Preparation

You can't succeed at the elimination protocol unless you put some time into planning and preparation. Prior to starting this protocol, you should spend a week getting ready. Start by greatly reducing or even eliminating some of the more common fibromyalgia problem foods: refined sugar, highly processed or fried foods, caffeine, red meat, MSG, aspartame, and alcohol. Use the preparatory week to wean yourself off caffeine so that you don't suffer withdrawal symptoms once you start the protocol.

Stocking Up on Groceries

Prior to the three weeks of the elimination phase of the protocol, you may need to stock up on a few things to keep meals interesting.

Good items to have in your pantry and fridge before starting include:

- organic rice milk (plain)—similar to skim milk in consistency; comes in boxes that can stay unrefrigerated for months; useful in cooking or for drinking straight.
- almond milk—another milk substitute with a nutty, sweet flavor; more like the consistency of low-fat milk; comes in boxes that can stay unrefrigerated for months; useful in cooking or for drinking straight. Try to find one without carrageenan.
- coconut and/or palm oil—a mixture of monounsaturated and saturated fats; exceptionally stable (long shelf life); excellent for baking and medium- to high-heat cooking; highly nutritious.
- olive oil—first cold press; for low- or no-heat uses.
- grains—millet, amaranth, quinoa, buckwheat. Get some of each and try them; you may find you have a new favorite grain!
- dry beans/legumes—lentils (red and green), kidney beans, black beans, pinto beans, navy beans, garbanzo beans (chickpeas).
- nuts and seeds—almonds, walnuts, hazelnuts, pine nuts, flax-seeds, sesame seeds, sunflower seeds. All should be raw and kept in the freezer.
- cans, boxes, or jars—tomato puree, crushed or chopped toma-toes, olives, artichoke hearts, green chilies, organic free-range chicken broth, vegetable broth without sugar.
- almond butter—raw and unsalted.
- tahini or sesame butter—raw and unsalted.
- herbal teas—there is an enormous selection of teas and tea blends available now that are delicious hot or cold. If you are quitting coffee, try slowly reducing your coffee grounds and substituting Teeccino until you are only using the Teeccino. This product comes in a few different flavors. You brew it like coffee, and it has more body than most teas. Another coffee alternative is Inka or other roasted chicory blends.

Open your calendar, and dedicate part of one day each week to menu planning and shopping for that week. Make note of any special occasions involving food for which you may need to plan ahead. As you get started, you'll want to track your meal planning, grocery lists, and favorite recipes in your Progress Journal. Talk to friends or family members who may follow special diets, and find out where they shop. Some grocery stores, such as Whole Foods, make it much easier to shop by providing a wide array of delicious gluten-free, dairy-free, and sugar-free (and artificial sweetener–free) products. Invest in a gluten-free or dairy-free cookbook, and search for recipes online. You'll find more helpful suggestions in the resources section of this book.

As you plan your menu, use the food lists and the sample menu here to help make decisions about what to eat. The foods that are off-limits include foods known to cause digestive problems, most IBS problem foods, typical allergens, inflammatory foods, and other foods known to cause symptoms commonly found in people with fibromyalgia. Don't panic. There are actually still plenty of foods you can eat, even if it means they aren't the same foods you usually eat. Check out the recipe section in the back of this book for additional ideas. If you have been diagnosed with IBS, you should also eliminate garlic, coconut, all nuts, and vegetables in the nightshade family (tomatoes, potatoes, onions, garlic, bell peppers, and eggplant), as these are common triggers of IBS.

Foods to Eat

Fruits and Vegetables

Unsweetened, dried fruit in moderation
All fresh fruit except citrus
All fresh or steamed vegetables except peas and corn

Protein

Chicken (unbasted; not processed; no antibiotics, hormones, colorings, etc.)
Turkey (unbasted; not processed; no antibiotics, hormones, colorings, etc.)
Fish (only wild; no antibiotics, hormones, colorings, etc.)
Nuts and nut butters (not peanuts)
Tahini (sesame butter)
Seeds (pumpkin, sunflower, etc.)
Beans, lentils, and other legumes (not peanuts)

Grains

Wild or brown rice
Quinoa, millet, amaranth, buckwheat

Sweeteners

Stevia

Beverages

Rice and almond milk without carrageenan or sugar (including rice syrup)
Herbal teas
Water
Vegetable juice (except carrot)

Foods to Eliminate

Dairy (milk, cheese, yogurt, butter, cream, ice cream) and "creamers"

Soy (tofu, soy milk, soy sauce, tamari, other soy products)

Peanuts (including peanut butter and peanut oil)

Wheat and yeasted foods (bread, pastries, pasta)

Corn (including oil, corn starch, syrup, maize, harina)

Gluten (wheat, barley, oats, rye, triticale, semolina, spelt, kamut, bulgur)

Shellfish

Eggs

Sugar, jams, jellies, honey, molasses, maple syrup

Highly processed or fried foods

Caffeine (tea; regular and decaffeinated coffee; soda, including diet soda)

Chocolate

Citrus (orange, grapefruit, lemon, lime)

Strawberries

Red meat, all processed meats (lunch meats, bacon, sausage, etc.)

MSG (monosodium glutamate)

Aspartame, Splenda, Equal, NutraSweet, saccharine, sorbitol, and other sugar alcohols

Black and red pepper

Alcohol (all alcohol, including wine and beer)

For IBS: Also exclude tomatoes, potatoes, eggplant, bell peppers, onions, and garlic

The Elimination Protocol

If you prepare carefully, the protocol won't be difficult to follow. In fact, it can feel very empowering to know you are doing something so beneficial for your health. Be sure to plan all your meals ahead so you don't get caught in a situation where you have to eat off-limit foods. The elimination protocol provides a great opportunity to explore new foods and leave your old eating habits behind. Take the time to be creative with this protocol—it doesn't have to be boring or bland. Also, be sure to drink lots of water. I recommend a minimum of 2 quarts a day: one before lunch and one before dinner. Each quart is equal to four glasses (8 oz.) of water. Carefully track all the food you eat in your Progress Journal, and make note of how you feel each day. It may take a week before you start to notice any significant improvement.

The first week of the elimination protocol will be the hardest. You may experience headaches and feel additional fatigue as your body protests about the changes in your diet. In the beginning, you may crave many of the foods that are off-limits. Your body is used to these foods, and as is the case with sugar and caffeine, may even be addicted to them. Your cravings will slowly diminish as the protocol progresses. Your taste buds, which have been bombarded with sugar for years, will regain their sensitivity, and seemingly ordinary foods will taste delicious. At the end of three weeks, you won't even want some of the foods that seem so hard to give up right now. You'll also be able to start rewarding yourself by reintroducing certain foods. Listed below are some sample menu ideas. These menu suggestions are easy to make, rely primarily on commonly used foods, and introduce some different and delicious foods. The resources section of this book suggests a cookbook, and the recipe section offers more delicious recipes.

Breakfast Ideas

When you wake up, you have not eaten for eight hours or more. Your body needs a combination of protein, carbohydrates, and healthful fat to prepare for the day. Many people experience their worst fibromyalgia symptoms in the morning. Starting your day with a healthful breakfast may help alleviate some of your symptoms and provide you with sustained energy and improved mental clarity. Here are a few breakfast options:

- Cooked millet or buckwheat with fresh or frozen berries and walnuts (hot or cold)
- Cooked quinoa and organic rice milk with fruit and sunflower seeds (hot or cold)
- Fresh fruit with almond milk (without carrageenan) and hazelnuts
- Smoothie with organic frozen fruit (no citrus) and coconut milk (rice protein powder is okay, but read the ingredients)
- Rice cakes with almond butter and fruit
- Buckwheat pancakes (be sure no wheat is in the mix) with fruit puree
- Amaranth cooked in almond milk with cinnamon and walnuts

Lunch or Dinner Ideas

An easy way to cut down on food-preparation time is to cook enough food at dinner to allow for lunchtime leftovers. To supplement your lunch, try fresh fruit, carrots, and celery.

- Chicken vegetable soup (without corn or peas) (see recipe section)
- Baked chicken with rice and steamed greens with fresh grated ginger
- Mixed green salad with veggies, sunflower seeds, and baked chicken. Dress with olive oil and balsamic vinegar.

- Baked wild Alaska salmon with wild rice and steamed broccoli with gomasio (sesame seeds and sea salt mixed together)
- Roast turkey breast with a sweet potato and green salad with vinaigrette dressing (see recipe section)
- Chicken and vegetable kebabs with brown rice and organic spinach sautéed in olive oil
- Grilled turkey breast with basil pesto, mashed sweet potato, and cauliflower
- Lentil dal with mochi (glutinous rice cake) and salad with olive oil–wine vinegar dressing
- Chili with ground turkey and brown rice (see recipe section)
- Cajun red beans and rice with kale and beets
- Wild rice–stuffed acorn squash with coconut oil and cinnamon
- Chicken and vegetable stir-fry over brown rice
- Roasted green chili, chicken, and white bean soup (see recipe section)
- Purple cabbage salad (see recipe section)

Snack Ideas

Be prepared by storing healthful snacks at your workplace, in your car, in your briefcase or purse, and in your gym bag. A healthful snack can keep your energy levels up and keep your metabolism from swinging to extremes. Having a little bit of healthful fat in your snack will help you feel full. Try these healthful snacks:

- Celery, jicama, or rice cakes with almond butter or hummus (see recipe section)
- Carrots and celery with almond butter

- Rice cakes with olive and artichoke tapenade (see recipe section)
- Raw almonds or walnuts
- Apple slices with almond butter
- Rice crackers with guacamole (see recipe section)
- Mochi (Grainaissance brand varieties that are acceptable are Original, Pizza, and Super Seed)

Beverages

- Water, water, water, water, water ...
- Herbal tea
- Rice milk (organic plain Rice Dream)
- Almond milk (without carrageenan or sugar)
- Vegetable juice (except carrot)
- Fruit juice (occasionally)

Sample Five-Day Menu

Make it easy on yourself. Follow this sample menu for the first five days. After that, mix and match from the recipe suggestions above, or come up with your own dishes.

Day 1

Breakfast: Fresh fruit with almond milk and hazelnuts
Lunch: Purple cabbage salad (see recipe section)
Dinner: Chili with ground turkey and brown rice (see recipe section)

Day 2

Breakfast: Rice cakes with almond butter and fruit
Lunch: Leftover chili
Dinner: Baked wild Alaska salmon with wild rice and steamed broccoli

Day 3

Breakfast: Buckwheat pancakes with fruit puree
Lunch: Fresh salad with avocado and turkey (olive oil and vinegar dressing)
Dinner: Roasted green chili, chicken, and white bean soup (see recipe section)

Day 4

Breakfast: Smoothie with frozen fruit (no citrus) and coconut milk
Lunch: Leftover chicken and white bean soup and/or Caesar salad (substitute cider vinegar for lemon juice)
Dinner: Chicken and vegetable kebabs with brown rice and organic spinach sautéed in olive oil

Day 5

Breakfast: Amaranth cooked in almond milk with cinnamon and walnuts
Lunch: Chicken and vegetable soup (see recipe section)
Dinner: Chicken and vegetable stir-fry over brown rice

The Challenge Phase

Once you have successfully completed three weeks on the elimination protocol, you can start to challenge your body by reintroducing each of the potential problem foods one at a time. Reintroduce no more than one new food category over a three-day period. You can choose the order in which you reintroduce the foods. It may take up to two days to notice the symptoms of food intolerance, which is why it is important to allow several days between reintroducing foods. You may not notice a food intolerance until you consume enough of that food to trigger symptoms. Caffeine (tea; regular and decaffeinated coffee; and soda, including diet soda), chocolate, sugar, red meat, and alcohol are particularly problematic for people with fibromyalgia, and I have not included them on the reintroduction list below. However, should you decide to reintroduce these foods to your diet, simply add them to the end of the following list:

1. Dairy (milk, cheese, yogurt, butter, cream, ice cream) and "creamers"
2. Gluten (wheat, barley, oats, rye, triticale, semolina, spelt, kamut, bulgur) and yeasted foods (bread, pastries, pasta)
3. Eggs
4. Soy (tofu, soy milk, soy sauce, tamari, other soy products)
5. Corn (including corn oil, corn starch, maize)
6. Citrus (orange, grapefruit, lemon, lime)
7. Strawberries
8. All processed meats (lunch meats, bacon, sausage, etc.)
9. Black and red pepper
10. Shellfish
11. Peanuts

If you have eliminated additional IBS problem foods (onions, garlic, tomatoes, potatoes, bell peppers, and eggplants), you should reintroduce them following the same systematic process. Keep in mind that IBS, like fibromyalgia, is a complicated illness. You may successfully reintroduce a food only to discover that it causes you problems later, perhaps because of the amount consumed or because it was consumed with a combination of foods that served to trigger an IBS episode.

Continue to record the food you eat and any symptoms that might occur in your Progress Journal. If you experience increased symptoms as you reintroduce a food, you need to consider whether the symptoms might have been caused by stress or another fibromyalgia trigger. Stop eating that particular food, and try introducing it on another occasion. If you experience similar symptoms, you should avoid that food. If you don't experience any symptoms after the introduction of a food, you can keep this food as part of your menu.

There is a good chance that as you reintroduce foods, you will continue to feel better and will not experience any additional symptoms. Consider yourself lucky if you do not have any obvious reactions to specific foods. Under these circumstances, any improvement in your health is due to the elimination of the fibromyalgia problem foods (sugar, alcohol, caffeine, red meat) in combination with a diet full of healthful and nutritious foods. If you do discover a problem food, modify how you eat accordingly. Once you have recovered from fibromyalgia, you may want to try a careful reintroduction of the problem food. There's a good chance it won't bother you when your sensations are no longer amplified.

Eating for Health

After you follow the elimination/challenge diet, you'll have a much better idea of how what you eat can affect how you feel. Once you've finished with the challenge portion of the elimination protocol, it is important to continue to eat a healthful and well-balanced diet. Your body needs a steady supply of essential nutrients, vitamins, and minerals to maintain your physical and mental health. As you have already discovered, this is especially true when you have fibromyalgia.

Let's face it—over the past hundred thousand years, our bodies have evolved without exposure to fast-food drive-thrus, call-in pizzerias, microwave dinners, vending-machine lunches, Big Gulps, or venti-sized lattes. As hunter-gatherers, we had to move to find our food. In the not-so-distant past, humans burned almost as many calories to catch, gather, and prepare the day's food as they took in from eating it. Our ancestors ate unprocessed, fresh, natural foods full of the vitamins and nutrients needed to keep up with the daily demands of survival. Today, we are able to consume a tremendous number of nutritionally empty calories with hardly any effort at all— just the opposite of what we actually need to stay healthy. So what should you be eating to give your embattled body a helping hand?

Carbohydrates, proteins, fats, vitamins, and minerals are the fundamental ingredients of a healthy diet. Beyond that straightforward fact, there is a huge array of often-contradictory information about nutrition in today's media marketplace. Many of my new patients are so confused about what type of diet they should follow that most of them have already thrown up their hands in defeat. If you're one of those people, read on. First, throw out all the fad diet books you have. These diets are not designed for your individual biochemistry, nor do they consider the special dynamics of fibromyalgia. Next, try to put the U.S. Department of Agriculture Food Pyramid, counting calories, and nearly everything you've heard about dietary fats out of your mind for the time being.

Unfortunately, there is simply no diet that works for everyone. In general, if you currently eat a typical American diet, you should do the following:

- Dramatically increase your intake of vegetables.
- Moderately increase your intake of fruits.
- Reduce your intake of fats in general, and limit yourself to healthy fats.
- Dramatically reduce your intake of simple carbohydrates.
- Eat lean meats and fish.
- Drink a lot more water.

The main nutrient groups (carbohydrates, protein, and fats) are described below. I recommend having something from each group at every meal, because the absorption of nutrients often occurs at optimal levels when foods are combined. If you follow the advice in this chapter and eat healthy foods in sensible portions, you will probably resolve any diet-related problems you are currently experiencing. The different nutrient groups are explained below, along with advice on the best foods to eat from each of these categories. Recommendations regarding caloric intake and specific proportions of food groups vary greatly according to an individual's metabolism, activity level, and digestive system, among other factors. The resources section at the end of this book provides a list of references for additional information. For more help on planning a diet that's right for your body, I recommend consulting a clinical nutritionist. See the resources section for more information on how to find a qualified clinical nutritionist.

Carbohydrates

Carbohydrates can be confusing because they constitute a *huge* grouping of foods. Carbohydrates are found in all fruits, vegetables, grains, and sugars, and everything made with these ingredients. The important thing to remember is that all carbohydrates contain components that eventually break down into glucose (blood sugar) in your body. As we've already discussed, complex carbohydrates break down slowly, while simple carbohydrates break down quickly, triggering a rapid rise in blood glucose. The body can only store a small amount of glucose. Excess glucose can trigger processes that cause damage to various body systems. Having too much extra circulating glucose can also contribute to inflammation and may make fibromyalgia symptoms worse. If you understand the general makeup of carbohydrates, you can control their breakdown and help stabilize the release and utilization of glucose.

Carbohydrates are now ranked on a glycemic index, which indicates how quickly a particular food causes your blood sugar to rise. Carbohydrates with high scores break down quickly into glucose and include white bread, cookies, white potatoes, white rice, ripe fruits, some vegetables (cooked carrots and beets, for example), as well as most snacks and desserts. To avoid the insulin spike associated with carbohydrates that causes a rapid rise in blood sugar, you need to choose foods with a low to moderate glycemic rating. These generally include complex carbohydrates that are also high in fiber, which slows down the release of glucose, thus providing energy over an extended period. Foods with low to moderate glycemic ratings include whole-grain bread and pasta, wild and brown rice, apples, oranges, grapefruit, corn, beans, and yogurt. The following adjustments to your diet can help reduce fatigue, increase your energy, help you lose weight, and improve your overall health as you work toward recovery:

- Use products made with whole grains. This includes replacing white bread with whole-wheat or whole-grain bread, switching from white to brown or wild rice, and using whole-grain cereals.
- Eliminate products with a high sugar content. This includes cakes, cookies, candy bars, brownies, cinnamon rolls, and other processed products generally made with refined white flour and loads of sugar.
- Try to eat some protein and healthy fat at every meal. This will help reduce any blood sugar swings brought on by carbohydrates by slowing down their conversion to glucose.

The University of Sydney has a searchable online database of different foods and their glycemic ratings. Do your own research at http://www.glycemicindex.com.

Protein Power

Protein consists of amino acids that build, maintain, and repair tissues in the body, including muscle. Proteins are also utilized to move nutrients and waste products into and out of cells and help to make it possible for fat-soluble substances to travel through the bloodstream. Eating good protein sources is vital as you regain energy and begin to rebuild your strength, and you should eat some at every meal. Anyone who eats a healthful, well-balanced, omnivorous diet will consume enough protein. Meat, vegetables, dairy, nuts, seeds, and grains all contain protein. However, like excess carbohydrates, excess protein will also be transformed into fat and stored in body tissue. The trick is to carefully choose the protein you eat. The easiest and most obvious sources of protein are animal products, but these are often high in saturated fat and cholesterol. Remember, it is best to eat red meat only on limited occasions. Healthful sources of protein include the following:

- wild salmon*
- seafood
- skinless chicken and turkey (choose lean, minimally processed meats)
- beans and lentils
- nuts and seeds
- dairy products (choose low-fat products)
- whole grains
- soy products

Fat Facts

Despite the bad rap it gets, fat is actually an important part of your diet. In addition to providing you with energy, fat is also required for the absorption and distribution of vitamins A, K, D, and E. It is the fat content of a meal that triggers satiety—meaning your brain gets the signal that you are full when a certain amount of fat makes it into your system. Without fats in a meal, you can end up eating far more calories and still feel hungry because the brain has not gotten the signal to shut

---

*Fresh, wild salmon is an excellent source of protein that is also high in healthful omega-3 oils. Farm-raised salmon are fed a grain diet that dramatically changes the fat-type ratios of the fish, which can have negative health impacts for humans nearly identical to those associated with consuming conventionally grown beef. A word of caution—wild fish can accumulate environmental toxins. Wild salmon can be safely consumed twice a week. Farm-raised salmon contain significantly higher levels of environmental toxins than wild fish and should be avoided.

off the hunger pangs. Too much fat can also be problematic, especially if you are consuming the wrong types of fat. And, as noted earlier, foods with a high fat content can also cause digestive problems, especially if you also suffer from IBS. Therefore, it is important for people with fibromyalgia to pay particular attention to the types of fats they consume.

Dietary fats are categorized as damaged fats, *trans*-fats, unsaturated fats, and saturated fats. Damaged fats comprise a category to strictly avoid. These can be found in deep-fried foods, many fast foods, junk foods, and any fat that has become rancid. *Trans*-fats negatively impact your health on many levels, including causing elevated and poorly balanced cholesterol levels, an increased risk of heart disease, and an increased risk of some cancers. Although *trans*-fats naturally occur in small quantities, most of the *trans*-fats you consume are created by the food industry through hydrogenation. Hydrogenation involves putting oil through a chemical process to make it hard or semihard at room temperature, like margarine. Food manufacturers must now identify *trans*-fats on food labels. Look for it in snack foods, baked goods, and fried foods. In contrast, unsaturated fats (poly- and mono-) are linked to good cholesterol levels and are found in sunflower, corn, soybean, canola, peanut, and olive oils. Saturated fats are more closely linked to health problems than are unsaturated fats, but they can be consumed in moderation. Healthful saturated fat is found in meat, milk, yogurt, butter, coconut, and palm oils. Saturated fats should be consumed in moderation, as large amounts are still linked to unhealthful cholesterol levels. Sources of healthy fats (unsaturated and saturated) include the following:

- olives/olive oil (unsaturated)
- coconut and palm oils (the only oils that should be used for medium- to high-heat cooking) (saturated)

- organic butter (saturated)
- avocados (unsaturated)
- walnuts, cashews, almonds, and their butters (both saturated and unsaturated fats)
- wild, cold-water, fatty fish (unsaturated)

For more information on nutrition, check out The Nutrition Source, a Web site maintained by the Harvard University School of Public Health: http://www.hsph.harvard.edu/nutritionsource.

Pure and Simple: Water

The simplest thing you can do to improve your diet and health is drink more water—as clean and pure as you can get. Most people are chronically dehydrated because they drink caffeinated beverages in place of water. Caffeine is a diuretic, meaning that it increases urine production and removes water from your system, exacerbating the dehydration problem. The body needs water to function efficiently on every level. The symptoms of even mild dehydration are extremely similar to some of your fibromyalgia symptoms:

- reduced metabolism
- daytime fatigue
- decreased cognitive abilities
- increased allergies
- muscle weakness
- headaches

In order to eliminate the chance that any of your symptoms are caused by dehydration, drink at least eight to ten 8-ounce glasses of water a day.

Vitamins, Minerals, and Other Supplements

Desperate to feel better, many fibromyalgia patients spend hundreds of dollars each year on vitamins, minerals, and other supplements. Although some of these may be helpful, others are a waste of money. The best way to ensure that your body has an adequate supply of vitamins, minerals, and nutrients is to eat a well-balanced diet that contains a variety of real, whole foods. In most cases, you should probably supplement your diet with a good food-based multivitamin. There are also some basic vitamins, minerals, and other supplements that may help improve your symptoms. I've summarized below the ones that are most likely to help fibromyalgia patients. I've also listed common foods you can use to obtain these vitamins, minerals, and other nutrients naturally.

Taking vitamin and mineral supplements is not always as straightforward as it might seem. For example, in order for your body to absorb iron, it needs to be taken with vitamin C. On the other hand, large doses of vitamin C can interfere with the absorption of vitamin B_{12}, so these two vitamins may need to be taken at separate times of the day. It is also important to buy a product that your body can readily absorb. For example, the body can absorb the calcium found in supplements containing calcium citrate more readily than those containing calcium carbonate. You can find additional information on vitamins, minerals, supplements, and a host of health-related issues at www.wholehealthmd.com and www.medlineplus.gov. The University of Maryland's Center for Integrative Medicine also posts valuable information on supplements at www.umm.edu/altmed/index.html. If you are unsure of how to best supplement your diet, it is always a good idea to work with a clinical nutritionist or medical doctor who is well-versed in nutrition.

If you decide to use other types of supplements, do your research carefully. Prescription drugs and over-the-counter (OTC) medications are tested and regulated by the Food and Drug Administration. Supplements are not regulated, but their potential side effects should still be taken seriously. Like drugs, many supplements need to be taken with the advice of a professional. If you are currently taking any prescription or OTC medications, check with your doctor before adding additional supplements. Some supplements and botanicals are known to interact poorly with prescription drugs or even other supplements.

If you do use supplements, be sure you are buying a quality product. Although many products are marketed as being formulated specifically for patients with fibromyalgia, they are no more specific to fibromyalgia than the vitamins or minerals you can find in any grocery store. The only real difference is the label and the price. The following Web sites have excellent information on herbal supplements, including which supplements interact poorly with different medications: www.wholehealthmd.com, www.medlineplus.gov, and www.herbmed.org. Be sure to make note of any vitamins or supplements you are taking in your Progress Journal.

Some of the supplements listed below are identified as antioxidants. Two recent studies suggest there may be a disruption in the oxidant/antioxidant balance in fibromyalgia patients. Oxidation in the body is a natural process resulting in highly unstable molecules known as free radicals. Free radicals are thought to sometimes fight off invading cells, but they are also known to damage the body's own cells. Antioxidants neutralize this process and are believed to play a role in boosting immune function and reducing the risk of chronic disease. Fresh fruits and raw vegetables are the best natural sources of antioxidants in your diet.

Multivitamin and Mineral Complex

A high-quality, food-based multivitamin helps maintain overall health by delivering a combination of minerals and vitamins. In the past, a balanced diet might have offered a complete range of vitamins and minerals, but in today's world of increasing toxin loads and depleted soils, even a diet composed solely of fresh, natural foods may be borderline deficient in some nutrients. If your diet is composed primarily of processed foods, the chances are even greater that mild to moderate nutrient deficiencies will develop.

Precaution: Multivitamins should be taken with food. Use a quality product; multivitamins contain many different ingredients, and quality control can be difficult. Check with your doctor or nutritionist to help determine the right multivitamin for you. Keep in mind that, in general, the cheaper the product, the cheaper the ingredients used to make it. The cheapest forms of certain nutrients may not be readily absorbed or utilized by your body.

Water-Soluble Vitamins

Vitamins B and C are water-soluble, which means that they dissolve in water and are not stored by the body, as fat-soluble vitamins are. As a result, vitamins B and C need to be replenished on a daily basis through diet and/or supplementation.

B Vitamins

B vitamins are fragile. They have a short shelf life in fresh foods and begin to deteriorate immediately after the fruit or vegetable is picked. They are also susceptible to damage or destruction via cooking methods and from prescription and OTC medications. Additionally, fight-or-flight chemicals destroy B vitamins quickly. If you have fibromyalgia, taking a B-complex vitamin might be a very good idea. B vitamins may help reduce the effects of stress and improve muscle weakness and fatigue by supporting the neuromuscular system. Low levels of vitamin B_{12} and folic acid are also associated with depression and may even reduce the effectiveness of certain antidepressants. B vitamins are found naturally in leafy green vegetables, asparagus, beans, citrus fruits, eggs, and dairy products.

Suggested Dose: B complex 50–100 mg per day

Precautions: Take with food to avoid nausea. Some people are sensitive to the energizing properties of B vitamins, so they should be taken with breakfast, not in the evening. If you are also supplementing with vitamin C, take the two vitamins at least two hours apart, as high doses of C will destroy some of the B vitamins. Folic acid, often found in B-complex vitamins, can interfere with certain antiseizure medications.

Note: The highly pigmented B vitamins that your body doesn't absorb are removed quickly by the kidneys. For this reason, don't be alarmed if your urine is bright yellow.

Vitamin C

Vitamin C bolsters the immune system and protects your body against infection. Vitamin C is essential for the regulation of neurotransmitters and also supports the adrenal glands. Chronic stress or infection may result in a depletion of vitamin C. This vitamin's antioxidant properties are especially important for fibromyalgia patients. Vitamin C helps with the absorption of iron, vitamin E, and other vitamins and minerals. Vitamins C, E, and glutathione are interdependent, acting to revitalize each other to maximize their antioxidant activities. Vitamin C is found in fruits and vegetables, especially oranges, orange juice, grapefruits, strawberries, tomatoes, and raw spinach.

Suggested Dose: 500–1000 mg per day in divided doses of 250 mg each throughout the day

Fat-Soluble Nutrients

Fat-soluble nutrients dissolve in fat and are absorbed into the bloodstream. They can be stored in the body longer than water-soluble vitamins but are not created by the body and so must be ingested either via diet or supplementation or both. Dietary fiber binds with lipids in the digestive tract, so if you are supplementing your diet with fiber or eating a high-fiber meal, take these nutrients two hours after eating with a small amount of nonfibrous, fatty food.

Coenzyme Q10

Coenzyme Q10 (CoQ10) is a supplement popular with many fibromyalgia patients. Its primary functions are to act as a part of the energy-producing apparatus in each cell in the body and to function as a key waste-removal molecule during energy production. Levels of CoQ10 have been shown to fall naturally over the life span but dramatically in energy depletion–related conditions and due to certain medications (such as the cholesterol-lowering statins). In 2002, a pilot study looked at the effects of giving CoQ10 (200 mg) and ginkgo biloba (200 mg) to fibromyalgia patients for eighty-four days. The study participants rated their quality of life as improved at the end of the study. However, this was a preliminary study that did not use a control group, so further testing is needed. Foods containing CoQ10 include fish and meat, with the highest amounts occurring in organ meats.

Suggested Dose: 30–100 mg twice per day of pharmaceutical-grade, all-*trans* CoQ10 in a lipid base

Precaution: There are huge numbers of poor-quality CoQ10 supplements on the market. Because CoQ10 is fat soluble, it must be taken in a gel-caplet form. Powders are useless. The type that has been shown to be most effective is naturally formed through a fermentation process. This form is identical to what the body makes. Chemically created CoQ10 is derived from tobacco. Consult a nutritionist or medical doctor well versed in nutrition about which brands are worth taking.

Vitamin D

Recent studies show that a vitamin D deficiency may be linked to muscle pain, low energy, fatigue, and mood swings. A vitamin D deficiency could certainly exacerbate your fibromyalgia symptoms. The body creates its own vitamin D from a modified cholesterol molecule when the molecule is exposed to sunlight through the skin. However, in northern latitudes (above latitude 40° north—in the United States, this region runs from just below New York City west to northern California), the sun is only strong enough to trigger the vitamin D conversion between May and September, and only if you are in the sun for at least fifteen to twenty minutes a day without sunscreen. If you are taking medications that interfere with cholesterol production in the body (statins), this will reduce the levels of vitamin D your body makes. Foods that are good sources of vitamin D include vitamin D–fortified milk, salmon, mackerel, cod liver oil, fish liver oil, some breads and grains, and egg yolks.

Suggested Dose: 400–1000 IU per day in winter months or all year if sun exposure is limited

Precaution: Vitamin D is stored in the liver, and you can overdose on it. Do not take a supplement if you are meeting the sun exposure requirements. The best sources of supplemental vitamin D are found in high-quality, uncontaminated fish oils.

Vitamin E

Vitamin E may be important to fibromyalgia patients, as it is a key antioxidant involved in the metabolism of cells. Vitamin E has numerous benefits and may help protect the body from chronic disorders. Vitamin E occurs naturally in nuts, seeds, leafy green vegetables, vegetable oil, wheat germ, and eggs. Vitamin C helps increase the absorption of vitamin E.

Suggested Dose: Vitamin E has two general classes: tocopherols and tocotrienols. Both groups have important but different antioxidant properties. Take 400 IU mixed natural tocopherols and tocotrienols daily with vitamin C.

Precaution: Avoid the synthetic forms of vitamin E by choosing products containing natural tocopherols and tocotrienols. High doses (over 800 mg) may interfere with blood clotting and the absorption of vitamin A. Vitamin E can act as a blood thinner and should not be taken in large doses the day prior to surgery and until surgical wounds have closed. Caution should be taken if you have high blood pressure or are taking blood pressure medication.

Essential Fatty Acids—Omega-3

Omega-3 essential fatty acids are converted into natural anti-inflammatory substances that help relieve the pain associated with inflammation. If you suffer any inflammatory conditions in addition to fibromyalgia, omega-3 fatty acids may reduce your discomfort. Omega-3 fatty acids may be particularly helpful for people who suffer from such inflammatory diseases as lupus and rheumatoid arthritis, both of which are key fibromyalgia triggers. Omega-3 fatty acids are also linked to the improvement of depression, another condition often experienced by fibromyalgia patients. These acids are found in the oils of cold-water fish (wild salmon, not farmed), eggs labeled as containing omega-3, flaxseeds, walnuts, buffalo meat, and grass-fed beef (not corn-fed or "grain-finished"). Omega-3 is generally supplemented through fish oil capsules containing EPA (eicosapentaenoic acid) and DHA (docosahexaenoic acid). When supplementing with fragile oils, it is important to pair them with the lipid-soluble antioxidants mentioned above to protect them.

Suggested Dose: 650–1000 mg per day of fish oil high in EPA

Precaution: It's important to use quality fish oil that is free of toxins and has been properly handled. Keep it in a cool place, and use it prior to the expiration date. High doses of fish oil may act as a blood thinner, so follow the recommendations for vitamin E supplementation with regard to surgery.

Minerals

Like vitamins, minerals are essential in various metabolic processes, and even mild deficiencies can cause disruption in the body's ability to function properly. There are two minerals that are of particular interest for people with fibromyalgia.

Magnesium

Preliminary clinical studies indicate that magnesium, given with malic acid, can reduce fibromyalgia pain and tenderness. A proper balance of magnesium and calcium are required for proper muscle function. Magnesium promotes muscle relaxation and proper nerve function. Magnesium inhibits the nerve receptors linked to trigger-point pain. It is also essential in the body's production of serotonin, an important neurotransmitter associated with mood. A magnesium deficiency in fibromyalgia patients could exacerbate fibromyalgia symptoms. Magnesium is found in cereals, nuts, sunflower seeds, tofu, bananas, avocados, spinach, and hummus.

Suggested Dose: 150–250 mg of magnesium three times per day and 400–800 mg of malic acid three times per day. Malic acid, calcium, and protein aid in the absorption of magnesium.

Precaution: Magnesium citrate is most easily absorbed by the body. Magnesium is best taken in combination with calcium, biotin, malic acid, and vitamin D, with a meal that contains protein. High-dose magnesium supplements can cause diarrhea. Don't take magnesium with tetracycline antibiotics. Talk to your doctor first if you have kidney or heart disease. The benefits of an increased intake can take six weeks or more to be realized.

Zinc

Adequate amounts of zinc, a trace mineral, are essential for a strong immune system. Clinical trials provide strong evidence that zinc, in combination with vitamin C, reduces the symptoms and shortens the duration of respiratory tract infections, including the common cold. When you have fibromyalgia, it seems like you come down with every single cold that goes around. Supplementing with zinc may give your body a slight boost in fighting off colds by improving your immune system. Zinc also has anti-inflammatory properties and may be important in preventing osteoporosis. Seafood, eggs, meats, whole grains, nuts, and seeds contain zinc. Coffee (regular and decaf), phytic acid (found in grain fiber and soy products), and cow dairy interfere with the absorption of zinc.

Suggested Dose: zinc citrate 30 mg per day

Precaution: High doses of zinc (200 mg and above) are toxic, may actually suppress immune function, and may disproportionately decrease high-density lipoprotein (HDL) cholesterol ("good" cholesterol). Zinc inhibits the absorption of copper and iron. If you are also taking an iron supplement, take zinc separately. Prolonged use of zinc may cause you to require copper supplementation. Zinc supplementation may also decrease the absorption of antibiotics, so it is recommended that supplements containing zinc be taken at least two hours away from antibiotics.

Other Dietary Supplements

5-HTP (5-hydroxytryptophan)

The body normally produces its own supply of 5-HTP from tryptophan and uses 5-HTP to produce the neurotransmitter serotonin. Low serotonin levels are associated with depression and anxiety, both of which occur frequently in fibromyalgia patients. Adequate levels of serotonin enhance mood, promote sleep, and influence appetite. In clinical trials, 5-HTP improved symptoms for some fibromyalgia patients. Tryptophan is found in poultry, fish, and dairy products.

Suggested Dose: 50–100 mg three times per day. Start with a low dose (50 mg) and gradually increase if symptoms do not improve.

Precaution: Do not take 5-HTP without talking to your doctor first. Mild side effects, including nausea, constipation, bloating, and drowsiness, may occur. 5-HTP has many known negative interactions with a large variety of prescription and OTC medications. Some of these include prescription antidepressants, Saint-John's-wort, carbidopa (for Parkinson's disease), and other medications that raise serotonin levels, such as Ultram (tramadol), Imitrex (sumatriptan), and Ambien (zolpidem). 5-HTP should not be taken with some OTC cold medicines.

L-Tyrosine

Tyrosine, a naturally occurring amino acid, is a precursor to virtually all of the fight-or-flight chemicals. The body uses tyrosine to make epinephrine, norepinephrine, serotonin, and dopamine. Several studies conducted in demanding military situations have indicated that supplementation with tyrosine may help counter the prolonged effects of psychological and physical stress by restoring depleted fight-or-flight chemicals. No studies have been conducted with fibromyalgia patients. Natural sources of tyrosine include soy products, chicken, turkey, fish, almonds, avocados, bananas, and dairy products.

Suggested Dose: 500–1000 mg three times a day, taken thirty minutes before meals. Tyrosine works best when combined with a multivitamin and mineral complex because vitamins B_6, B_9 (folate), and copper help with the synthesis of L-tyrosine into the fight-or-flight chemicals.

Precaution: Consult with a knowledgeable healthcare provider prior to adding tyrosine to your diet. Tyrosine can trigger migraine headaches and gastrointestinal discomfort. Tyrosine may increase blood pressure when combined with monoamine oxidase inhibitors. Tyrosine should not be taken with the Parkinson's medication levodopa.

SAM-e (S-adenosylmethionine)

SAM-e contributes to the production of serotonin and dopamine, both of which are depleted in fibromyalgia patients. SAM-e has primarily been studied for its beneficial effects as an antidepressant. SAM-e also has anti-inflammatory and pain-reducing qualities. Clinical trials with fibromyalgia patients have provided evidence that SAM-e may be effective in improving mood and reducing pain, fatigue, and stiffness. The body normally produces its own supply of SAM-e.

Suggested Dose: 400 mg two times daily, increased to three times daily after three weeks if no improvement. Reduce dose to 200 mg two times per day once improvement begins.

Precaution: Consult with your doctor before taking SAM-e. SAM-e should not be taken with antidepressants or with levidopa (taken for Parkinson's disease).

Saint-John's-Wort

The supplement Saint-John's-wort is derived from a common shrub of the same name. Saint-John's-wort is clinically proven to alleviate the symptoms of mild to moderate depression and is commonly prescribed as an antidepressant in Germany. Saint-John's-wort is believed to work by elevating serotonin levels in the brain.

Suggested Dose: 450 mg two times per day with meals

Precaution: Saint-John's-wort may interact with some medications. Consult with your doctor before taking Saint-John's-wort with other medications. Saint-John's-wort should not be combined with other antidepressants or 5-HTP. Saint-John's-wort can cause photosensitivity, so be careful not to burn when outside in the sun. Results may take six weeks or more to be realized.

MSM *(methyl-sulfonyl-methane)*

MSM is widely reported to relieve the pain associated with arthritis and inflammatory conditions, and now clinical trials are confirming it. MSM occurs naturally in fresh fruits, rye, vegetables, and milk. MSM is often sold in combination with glucosamine and chondroitin.

Suggested Dose: 800–1200 mg per day

Glucosamine and Chondroitin

In combination, glucosamine and chondroitin may promote joint cartilage formation, repair, and elasticity. The deterioration of cartilage adversely impacts joints and leads to osteoarthritis.

The American College of Rheumatology recommends chondroitin for osteoarthritis treatment. Glucosamine has also been shown to slow the progression of osteoarthritis. Glucosamine and chondroitin may also help with other types of arthritis and joint-related conditions. There is no commonly available food source of glucosamine or chondroitin. Supplements are readily available.

Suggested Dose: glucosamine (500 mg three times per day); chondroitin (400 mg three times per day)

Precaution: Do not take chondroitin in combination with blood thinners or if you are also challenged with cancer in any form. Check with your doctor for potential drug interactions. It may take several months before you notice any benefits. Since most chondroitin is obtained from bovine (cow) cartilage, be sure you are getting a quality, toxin-free product.

How to Choose Supplements

1. Use caution with any supplement that claims to cure a multitude of ailments—if it sounds too good to be true, it probably is.

2. Look for "food-based" nutrients. These are generally easier for your body to recognize and assimilate than the laboratory-created versions.

3. Never buy lipid-based supplements (fish or flaxseed oil, CoQ10, etc.) in bulk, and always store them in a cool, dark place. Some may require refrigeration to maintain their integrity.

4. Buy only natural vitamin E supplements with the full range of eight tocopherols and tocotrienols.

5. Look for labels that give you detailed information on the molecular forms of each nutrient—for example, instead of just calcium, look for calcium citrate.

6. Realize that no single company or product line does everything well. You will want to research each supplement separately rather than choose a single brand. Look in the resources section of this book for more information on where to find information.

7. Work with a clinical nutritionist or MD who knows supplements, because he or she will recognize the quality brands. However, be wary of anyone who tells you that you must purchase all your supplements through him or her. A good practitioner will offer you a range of options to fill each particular supplement need, including the purchase of supplements elsewhere.

In a Nutshell . . .

- If you have fibromyalgia, certain foods may be causing or exacerbating some of your symptoms.
- Some common fibromyalgia problem foods are wheat, gluten, dairy, red meat, refined sugar, alcohol, MSG, aspartame, caffeine, fried food, and junk food.
- Problem foods can cause headaches, flulike symptoms, digestive problems, inflammation, blood sugar swings, dehydration, and even mood swings.
- Following an elimination diet can help you discover whether certain foods exacerbate your fibromyalgia symptoms.
- Eat a healthful, well-balanced diet that includes protein, carbohydrates, and fats at every meal.
- Eliminate simple, high-glycemic carbohydrates (sugar, bread, potatoes) and increase complex, low-glycemic carbohydrates (veggies, fruits, and whole grains).
- As you recover from fibromyalgia, you will once again be able to eat any of the foods you ate without problems before you developed fibromyalgia.
- Consider nutritional supplementation under the guidance of a healthcare professional well-versed in both nutrition and fibromyalgia.

CHAPTER 9

An Exercise Program That Helps *More Than It* Hurts

The mere mention of exercise to a group of fibromyalgia patients often elicits a flood of emotion and frustration:

> "Whenever I try to exercise, I can't get out of bed for the next three days."
>
> "Getting through the day takes all the energy I have. Exercise is out of the question!"
>
> "I am so tired of hearing about how I just need to exercise! I can hardly walk up the stairs."

If you have suffered from fibromyalgia for long enough, you are probably tired of being told that a little exercise will make you feel better. How many times have well-meaning friends, family, and even physicians and therapists instructed you to "do a little more" or "push yourself a little harder"? Don't they get it? Exercise hurts! If you had a broken leg, no one would tell you to go get some exercise. Unfortunately, you have an illness that keeps you looking healthy enough, your symptoms vary from day to day, and people can't seem to understand that you *really* are exhausted and it *really* does hurt when you do more than you should.

Exercise presents a double-edged sword for fibromyalgia patients. A lack of exercise leads to weight gain and muscle weakness, making your symptoms worse. On the other hand, attempts to exercise often result in increased pain, overwhelming fatigue, and tremendous frustration. Many people with fibromyalgia get stuck in this downward spiral and soon find that even the simplest of household chores are impossible. In light of all that, it may be hard to believe that regular exercise is an important part of your long-term recovery.

Movement is a form of medicine for your muscles, joints, tendons, and ligaments. Finding the right exercise program requires as much attention and effort as finding the right type and amount of medication. Like most medications, exercise needs to be done every day. The prescription is also different for everyone. An exercise program that helps one of my patients may actually create more problems for another. You need to find the right type and amount of exercise for your body so you feel better instead of worse. Now that you understand your own cycle of fibromyalgia, you are in a much better place to make exercise a key ingredient in your success story. Although exercise is important, keep in mind that it will probably take at least a month of exercising consistently to feel the benefits.

With exercise, the amount of time it takes to see results will vary for each person, because everyone will start at a different fitness level. However, if you stick to a program, I guarantee that you will see slow and steady results in terms of improved strength, flexibility, and energy level. This chapter will show you how to find a program that's right for you.

Problems with *Not* Exercising

Our bodies were designed for movement. We did not evolve to sit in front of computers all day, drive cars long distances, or otherwise function as couch potatoes. Exercise is an invention of the modern world—a necessity forced on us by the sedentary nature of society. Getting enough exercise is a problem for the vast majority of Americans. A lack of physical activity, in combination with poor eating habits, is one of the most pressing health problems in the country, leading to an increased risk of heart disease, diabetes, and hypertension. Although everyone has an excuse for not getting enough exercise, fibromyalgia patients face more than their share of obstacles. If you have tried exercise and have subsequently given up, you shouldn't feel bad or guilty.

The fibromyalgia cycle causes you to gradually become more sedentary in an effort to avoid pain and conserve energy. If you enjoyed a regular exercise regimen before developing fibromyalgia, the inability to exercise likely adds to your stress and frustration. Even if you didn't necessarily exercise before you had fibromyalgia, your activity level has probably still decreased measurably. The lack of exercise that often accompanies fibromyalgia creates a new set of problems for your body to contend with. As your activity level decreases, your muscles slowly lose their tone and conditioning.

Poorly conditioned muscles are more susceptible to injury from even mild activity, resulting in additional stress and strain on your body. Poorly conditioned muscles also use more energy to accomplish tasks, adding to your fatigue. Seemingly minor changes in your daily routine, such as reduced housecleaning or gardening, negatively affect your flexibility and range of motion. Most patients note tightness and knots developing in underused and poorly stretched muscles. These areas are generally very painful, and the tightness can spread throughout the body. The gradual cessation of such activities as preparing meals, walking the dog, taking the stairs, or cleaning up around the house contributes to a loss of flexibility and range of motion. A lack of exercise results in

- muscle atrophy
- loss of flexibility and range of motion
- increased susceptibility to injury
- fatigue
- loss of muscle function
- reduced physical function
- muscle knots and tension
- increased stiffness and soreness
- weight gain
- depression

Fibromyalgia patients struggle with finding enough energy to get through the day. Attempts to exercise can lead to increased exhaustion and pain. If you've tried exercise in the past and found that it seemed to make your symptoms worse, you might be afraid to try exercising again. Fortunately, there's an upside to exercise as well.

The Upside to Exercise

In general, people who exercise consistently lead healthier, happier, and longer lives. Exercise reduces pain, improves sleep, reduces tension, staves off depression, improves self-esteem, increases energy, contributes to weight loss, and keeps the body flexible and strong. The problem with fibromyalgia is that all of these big-picture benefits aren't so easily obtainable, because you need to start an exercise program more slowly and carefully than most other people. I consistently encounter fibromyalgia patients who wanted to exercise but tried to accomplish too much too soon, with devastating results. Researchers have spent a lot of time trying to determine whether exercise helps people with fibromyalgia. The most consistent and perhaps important clinical finding is that gentle aerobic exercise and/or carefully supervised strength training improve fitness and increase physical functioning in fibromyalgia patients.

What does this mean for you? It means that if you can follow an appropriate exercise program, you're likely to see the following results:

- Your strength and endurance will improve.
- You'll increase the number of tasks you can accomplish on a daily basis.
- Everyday chores that seem so difficult now will become more routine and less daunting. Depending on your fitness level when you start, your improvements may range from walking up the stairs without effort to enjoying a walk in the park.
- As your stamina improves, grocery shopping, gardening, and even working a day at the office may seem less demanding.
- Most important, you'll stop the downward spiral that takes place when decreased activity impairs muscle functioning and subsequently limits activity even more.

What about the effects of exercise on pain? Anyone who starts a new exercise program expects a certain amount of soreness after actively using muscles again. Most people describe this as a "good" sore, because they know it means they're getting stronger. There's no such thing as good sore for fibromyalgia patients. The typical pain and soreness that accompany a new exercise regimen can result in unbearably amplified pain signals. However, with a carefully designed program, you can successfully exercise without increasing your pain.

Clinical Findings—Exercise and Pain

Most people refrain from exercise because they're afraid of increasing their pain. It's true that inappropriate exercise will increase pain. However, in a wide variety of studies, researchers found that appropriate levels and types of exercise consistently produce benefits without increasing pain scores. On an even more positive note, multiple studies have found that exercise significantly reduces pain scores for fibromyalgia patients.

Exercise also plays an important role in your recovery by providing an outlet for an overactive fight-or-flight response. The message of the fight-or-flight response is one of motion— when the brain perceives a threat, adrenaline prepares the body for *action*. In today's world, the fight-or-flight response engages in situations where action isn't appropriate. The adrenaline running through your veins, encouraging you to take action, is at odds with your inability to use purely physical means to solve problems. Exercise provides one solution to this dilemma. Aerobic exercise mimics the action demanded by the fight-or-flight response. In turn, adrenaline levels dissipate and the sympathetic nervous system relaxes.

Set Yourself Up for Success

If you're ready to implement an exercise program, the following considerations will help ensure that your endeavor is a successful one:

- Choose an exercise you enjoy.
- Research the types of programs available.
- Determine the best time of day to exercise.
- Pay attention to your symptoms.
- Set realistic expectations.
- Make a commitment to yourself.

Choose an Exercise You Enjoy

The most important part of an exercise program is your ability to stick to it. You can greatly increase the odds of success by choosing an exercise you enjoy. If you choose an exercise that seems boring or tedious, you may find motivation hard to come by. Some people enjoy exercising alone, while others prefer group activities. If you can't find a suitable exercise that appeals to you, finding a group or an exercise partner may help keep you committed. Another good option is to combine exercise with something else you enjoy. For example, if you choose walking as an option, find a friend to keep you company as you walk. Books on tape are another great motivator. If you listen to an engaging book while you exercise, you may find yourself making excuses to exercise more often so that you can listen to one more chapter. (The trick is to refrain from listening to the book if you're not also exercising.) Keep in mind that the beginning of any exercise program is the hardest. Once you make exercise part of your routine, you will start looking forward to that part of your day.

Research the Types of Programs Available

If you don't want to exercise alone, spend some time researching the types of exercise programs available in your area. Your local hospital or YMCA is a good place to start, as many have programs specifically tailored for people with fibromyalgia. Programs designed for people with arthritis pain may also be suitable for your needs. Contact your local YMCA or senior center for a list of fitness programs tailored for people with physical challenges, such as arthritis or fibromyalgia. Local chapters of the National Arthritis Foundation organize exercise programs for people who have arthritis, including an aquatic exercise program. In order to find a chapter near you, contact the National Arthritis Foundation at 800-568-4045. You might also want to check with studios that specialize in yoga, tai chi, or Pilates for a program that meets your needs.

Determine the Best Time of Day to Exercise

When do you feel the best? If you feel good, you'll more easily find the motivation to exercise. If your schedule is flexible, time your exercise regimen to coincide with the part of the day when you're most likely to have some energy. This might not be as hard as you think. In the beginning, you may only exercise ten minutes per day. Depending on the type of exercise you choose, this may be easily incorporated into a mid-morning or lunch break. Also, if you know you will need rest after exercise, avoid planning back-to-back activities.

Pay Attention to Your Symptoms

Before you exercise, take a moment to assess how you feel that day. Are you rested? How is your energy level? Are your symptoms better or worse than they were the last time you exercised? If you're having a hard day, take a step back and do a little less. Progress doesn't always mean doing more. Some days, progress means knowing when to give your body a rest.

Set Realistic Expectations

Expectations are an important part of your fitness program. Take a moment to think about your pre-fibromyalgia fitness level.

_____ Total couch potato

_____ Minimal/occasional exercise

_____ Moderate/consistent exercise (2 to 3 times/week)

_____ Strenuous/consistent exercise (4 to 7 times/week)

_____ Total athlete

If you have previous experience with exercise, this will play a large role in determining how much you think you should be able to do. If you followed a regular exercise program or participated in athletic activities prior to developing fibromyalgia, you can use this experience to your advantage. You have already experienced the benefits of maintaining a healthy body through exercise. The disadvantage of your past experience is that you may set unrealistic expectations for yourself. You may also be easily bored by or frustrated with your inability to exercise at your pre-fibromyalgia level. There is no reason to push your body. High-intensity aerobic exercise has no benefits over low-intensity aerobic exercise for people with fibromyalgia. Picking the appropriate level and type of exercise will help minimize some of the short-term pain that may accompany increased activity. You should expect to have some pain and soreness in the beginning. As long as the pain is tolerable and short-term, continue exercising. After the initial period, any additional pain and soreness should disappear.

No matter how much you exercised in the past or how determined you are to regain strength, the key to success is making a slow start. In the beginning, always do less than you think you actually can. For many people, *this means adding just one extra thing per day*. For example, if you are currently stuck at home, your exercise may consist of simply walking to the corner on a daily basis. For someone who is more active, exercise may involve participating in a group class two or three times a week. If you choose to exercise with a group, do not expect to match the strength or endurance of other participants. If you try to compete with more experienced or healthier participants, you may injure yourself or aggravate your symptoms. When starting a new program, always discuss your fibromyalgia with the instructor prior to the first class.

You need to believe that someday, you will once again enjoy the level of activity you were used to before the fibromyalgia cycle started. In the meantime, readjust your expectations to the current reality of your life. To do otherwise might cause additional harm or injury to your body. Don't avoid exercise because you are afraid of or embarrassed by your current limitations. Accept where you are now, and work toward a healthier, stronger future.

Make a Commitment to Yourself

Exercise will yield improvements if done with consistency and discipline. Prior to starting any new endeavor, commit to at least six weeks of consistent exercise. Use a calendar to put your weekly goals in writing. Each time you exercise, make a note of your accomplishment in the calendar. You can also use your calendar to track changes in your symptoms and physical abilities. Although you may start slowly, your calendar will document your continued commitment to exercise.

Conduct a Self-Assessment

Next, you should determine the most effective amount of exercise for your body. The following questions are designed to help you assess your current physical abilities. The answers to these questions will help you develop a baseline against which you can measure future improvements. Although your symptoms may vary daily or weekly, choose your answers according to your most recent, consistent activity level.

Circle the letter that best describes your current condition:

    a) Avoid all exercise.
    b) Exercise periodically (1 to 3 times/month).
    c) Exercise on a semiregular basis (1 to 2 times/week).
    d) Exercise consistently (3 to 4 times/week).

Circle the letter that best describes your current condition:

    a) Walk with great difficulty or not at all.
    b) Able to walk three to five city blocks.
    c) Prefer to walk whenever possible.
    d) Walk whenever I can; climb stairs easily.

Circle the letter that best describes your current condition:

    a) Unable to perform most household chores.
    b) Able to perform easy chores (washing dishes, folding laundry, sweeping).

c) Able to perform moderate chores (vacuuming, watering plants, putting away pots and pans).

d) Able to perform difficult chores (cleaning out garage, mowing lawn).

Circle the letter that best describes your current condition:

a) Severe pain from fibromyalgia and/or other conditions, such as osteoarthritis, that consistently prevents me from engaging in everyday activities.

b) Moderate pain from fibromyalgia and other conditions, such as tendonitis, is aggravated by exercise or other activities.

c) Moderate pain from fibromyalgia slows me down but does not limit my activity.

d) Mild pain from fibromyalgia only—doesn't limit my activity.

Develop Your Own Exercise Program

Once you've taken the self-assessment, add up your points according to the following scale:

a = 1 point
b = 2 points
c = 3 points
d = 4 points

The recommendations below are based on the total number of points derived from the self-assessment. If you are uncertain of an answer or you cannot decide between different levels, choose the lower level. It is always safer to be conservative. These are guidelines only and are not a substitute for an exam from an experienced professional. If you have an underlying medical condition or concerns about your ability to perform any of the recommended exercises, consult with a physician or physical therapist prior to starting a program.

Level 1 (4–6 points)

If you received 6 points or fewer, I don't recommend a self-directed program. An extremely mild, modified exercise program may be appropriate when conducted under the supervision of a physical therapist or equivalent professional. I recommend focusing your recovery efforts in the other areas outlined in this book. Specifically, take the time to resolve any underlying medical causes, make sure you're getting quality sleep, and focus your efforts to control the fight-or-flight response. If you haven't already, follow the diet modifications outlined in chapter 8. You can also make modest efforts to increase strength and endurance through everyday activities.

Level 2 (7–10 points)

If your total equaled 7 to 10 points, you are ready to start a gentle exercise program with gradual increases in effort. The best activity for you is probably swimming or a water aerobics class designed for people with arthritis or fibromyalgia. These exercises will minimize the impact on your joints and muscles while allowing you to modestly increase strength, flexibility, and endurance. Contact local swimming pools or the YMCA for information on programs near you. If you are able to find a suitable water aerobics class, try to attend twice a week. Start by participating in the first ten to fifteen minutes of the class, and work your way up until you can stay for the entire class. If you choose swimming, start very slowly. If you only swim four laps on your first visit to the pool, that's still a great start. Try to swim three times a week.

Another good option for you is to develop a self-paced walking program. Start by walking less than you think you can. If you think you can walk for ten minutes, start by walking eight. Gradually increase the time you walk as it feels appropriate. If you want to incorporate some gentle stretching into your routine, follow the stretching guidelines at the end of this chapter. You might also find some specialized yoga or tai chi classes that are appropriate for you.

Level 3 (11–13 points)

If you scored 11 to 13 points, chances are you would benefit from a consistent exercise program designed to increase strength, flexibility, and endurance. Choose the aerobic exercise—swimming, walking, or cycling—that most appeals to you. Regardless of how good you feel, start with less exercise than you think you can do, and build up gradually. You can also mix and match exercises. You may want to swim one day a week and walk three days a week. In the beginning, try to engage in aerobic activity two to three times a week. As you feel better, follow the recommendations for the Level 4 exercise program and increase the amount you exercise to four to six days a week. You may also want to incorporate a yoga, tai chi, or Pilates class one to two times a week to improve your flexibility and core strength. You can also perform these exercises at home with the help of a video. Use great care not to overstretch your muscles during these exercises. Follow the stretching guidelines at the end of this chapter. As you feel stronger and are able to exercise more, retake the self-assessment to determine if your exercise program is improving your ability to perform daily activities.

Level 4 (14–16 points)

If you scored 14 to 16 points, you are likely at a point in the fibromyalgia cycle where exercise would be extremely beneficial. If you're already exercising consistently, you may want to slowly increase the amount of exercise you get each week. Start with the aerobic activity of your choice three to five times a week. If you haven't been exercising, start with less than you think you are capable of. If you think you can walk for thirty minutes with no problem, then walk for twenty minutes the first few times. Apply the same principle to swimming, cycling, or any other activity you engage in. You should ultimately exercise four to six days a week for thirty to sixty minutes each time. You may also want to incorporate a yoga, tai chi, or Pilates class one to two times a week to improve your flexibility and core strength. You can also perform these exercises at home with the help of a video. Use great care not to overstretch your muscles during these exercises. Follow the stretching guidelines at the end of this chapter.

Important Considerations

Know Your Body—Scores Are Only a Guide. The score from your self-assessment and the sample programs detailed for various exercise levels should serve as a guideline to get you started. You know the limits and special considerations of your body, and ultimately you will have to decide what type of exercise works best for you. If you have attempted to exercise in the past without success, carefully consider what might have gone wrong, and make adjustments as needed. In all cases, it would be wise to consult with a doctor, physical therapist, or trainer who has specialized knowledge on how to assist fibromyalgia patients with exercise.

Other Medical Conditions May Require You to Take Precautions. If you have another medical condition such as heart disease, osteoporosis, or a previous injury, you have a different set of circumstances to consider when starting any new exercise. If you're not familiar with the limitations of your other medical conditions, consult with your doctor or physical therapist before starting to exercise. These professionals will be able to tell you if there are certain activities you should stay away from or if there are modifications that can help you participate successfully in an exercise program.

Work with a Trainer or Instructor. Prior to starting any class or program, schedule time to talk with the instructor or trainer about your condition and any limitations you might have. If at all possible, it is best to work with someone who has experience working with fibromyalgia patients. Regardless of who you work with, you are the only one who will truly know when you should stop. The motto "no pain, no gain" simply does not apply to fibromyalgia patients. You should never let anyone encourage you to overexert yourself or push your outer limits. Instead, you should exercise within the confines of safely controlled parameters. If an exercise hurts or causes pain while you are doing it, then you're asking too much of your body. Although some residual soreness is normal, as discussed above, you should never be in pain while you are exercising.

Track Your Progress. Regardless of the type of exercise you choose, develop a system for setting goals and tracking your progress. Do not get caught up in comparing your performance from one session to another or even from the beginning of the week to the end. Most of my patients find that progress is slow, with peaks and valleys. Also realize that your progress may not show up as the ability to do more exercise.

It may be that you stay at the same level for several weeks but that you can now do more at home or with the kids.

You can use something similar to the sample chart below to write down your goals and track results in your Progress Journal. Writing down goals and developing your own exercise program will help you stay committed to consistent exercise. However, you should constantly reevaluate your goals and reassess your abilities. Don't be afraid to redefine your goals on a weekly basis. If you complete a week of training and are not feeling ready to move on, repeat the same week over again or step back a week, if necessary. It is important to have something to work toward, but you should not try to meet unrealistic goals at any cost. It is more important to move slowly and exercise consistently than it is to move too fast and then give up altogether.

WALKING PROGRAM

	Week 1—Goal: 15 minutes	Week 2—Goal: 18 minutes
Day 1	June 6—walked 10 minutes	June 13—walked 12 minutes
Day 2	June 7—felt mostly good; a little sore	June 14—no soreness
Day 3	June 8—walked 12 minutes	June 15—walked 15 minutes
Day 4	June 9—still a little sore, but better	June 16—felt good; just a little sore
Day 5	June 10—walked 12 minutes	June 17—walked 18 minutes
Day 6	June 11—felt good; no soreness	June 18—had more energy today

At the beginning of your program, make a list of the daily activities you can no longer take part in—everything from washing dishes to walking the dog. (See the Physical Activity Wish List and Tracking Your Progress worksheets at the end of this chapter.) As you proceed, use this list to measure your progress. Your physical abilities in daily life are a more important measure of progress than the distance you can walk, swim, or cycle.

Recommended Exercises

There are many different exercise possibilities for fibromyalgia patients to choose from. Your physical needs and personal preference are important criteria in choosing the right type of exercise for you. Research indicates that for fibromyalgia patients, gentle aerobic exercise consistently produces a greater number of benefits with fewer risks than does stretching or strength training. In this section, I'll describe the benefits of swimming/water exercise, walking, cycling, and a variety of nontraditional exercises, including yoga, tai chi, and Pilates. You are certainly not limited to choosing from the programs described in this chapter. However, I have deliberately focused on this subset of exercises because in my experience, these exercises provide the greatest benefits without aggravating symptoms.

Swimming or pool exercises, walking, and cycling are all low-impact exercises that produce aerobic benefits. If you have been sedentary for an extended period of time, your muscles need a gentle period of reconditioning that is easily achievable with any of these exercises. Each of these exercises will help improve your endurance, strength, and to some extent flexibility and range of motion. It is also easy to swim, walk, or cycle at your own pace and at the time of day that works best for you. If you prefer to exercise with a group or instructor, these exercises are readily available at a variety of locations. Many of my patients are also turning to yoga, tai chi, and Pilates as nonaerobic options that increase strength and flexibility and can be done at home or in a group setting. These activities often have a meditative aspect that helps ease stress and reduce anxiety.

Advantages of Walking, Swimming, or Cycling

- Low-impact exercise
- Not likely to aggravate symptoms
- Have proven benefits for fibromyalgia patients
- Available at your own time and pace
- Easily affordable

In the beginning, avoid such exercises as jogging, running, or high-impact aerobics. These exercises place more pressure on your joints and require a greater exertion of energy and a wider range of muscle movement. These exercises are more likely to result in injury and increased pain. Even the slightest degree of trauma to your muscles, joints, tendons, or ligaments may result in amplified pain signals that prevent the continuation of an exercise program. In the beginning, I recommend that you avoid weight training. Some of the muscle contractions required for weight training are extremely likely to cause muscle damage and increased pain. If you are interested in weight training, find a professional trainer familiar with the best ways to maximize benefits and reduce risks for people with fibromyalgia.

Swimming/Water Exercise

Swimming and doing water aerobics in a warm-water pool are ideal exercises for reducing fibromyalgia symptoms and increasing physical capacity. Most pool therapy takes place in water that is 85 to 86 degrees Fahrenheit, allowing the warm water to soothe the muscles and promote relaxation. When you enter a pool, the water helps support your weight and minimizes the stress typically placed on the joints and muscles during other types of exercise. Water also has a compressive force called hydrostatic pressure that helps decrease pain, reduce any swelling, and increase blood flow. Water provides a fairly consistent resistance to exercise through your entire range of motion. The faster you move, the more resistance you will face.

Exercising in water allows for great variability in your routine. You can walk in the pool at different depths and speeds to get different resistances, or you can perform range-of-motion exercises or strength exercises. Water makes it easy to stretch in weight-bearing and non-weight-bearing positions, and you can perform aerobic exercise with many different movement patterns, from jogging to jumping jacks. These are all excellent ways to improve your range of motion and flexibility without exacerbating your symptoms. If you have joint problems or suffer from osteoarthritis, pool-based exercises may be the best choice for you.

The benefits of pool exercise carry over to the land. Swimming or water aerobics will elevate your heart rate, improving your overall stamina and physical fitness. My patients who perform pool exercises often report rapid improvement in their cardiovascular capacity, the ability to walk faster and farther, and more of an energy gain than my patients who choose land-based exercise. The pool also seems to increase their sense of well-being, and many people report a reduction in pain, anxiety, and depression.

You can usually participate in water aerobics even if you don't know how to swim. These exercises may be held in the shallow end of the pool or with the use of flotation devices under supervision. Contact your local YMCA or health club for information on water aerobics classes. Many classes designed to help people with arthritis will also be suitable for people with fibromyalgia. If you know how to swim, a membership at an indoor swimming pool is your passport to regaining strength, flexibility, and self-confidence. When you start swimming, vary your strokes. Freestyle (the crawl), backstroke, and breaststroke will each gently stretch and strengthen different muscle groups. Even though swimming is a gentle exercise, you should start slowly and stop before you feel tired.

Clinical Findings

A twenty-week study compared the effects of pool-based exercise programs with land-based exercise programs for fibromyalgia patients. Both groups increased their cardiovascular capacity, improved measured walking times, and experienced less daytime fatigue. The pool-based group also experienced more "good" days and reported improvement in physical impairment, pain, anxiety, and depression. These results remained unchanged during a six-month follow-up period. Other studies have also reported positive results.

Walking

If you feel apprehensive about starting any type of fitness program, walking may be the perfect exercise for you. Walking doesn't require any special equipment, skills, or training. It can be done anytime, anywhere, and with anyone. It is easy to tailor a walking program to suit your needs—all you have to do is listen to your body. You don't need a trainer, therapist, or specialized program to incorporate walking into your daily routine.

Walking will yield the same aerobic benefits as swimming, although there is more risk of increased pain if you walk too fast or for too long. You do not have to walk fast. Walking at a comfortable pace yields more beneficial results for fibromyalgia patients. Walking fast, long distances, or on inclines will cause more pain initially and make it harder for you to continue your exercise program. If you have access to a gym or home treadmill, this may be the safest way to start walking, as the treadmill will provide more cushion for your joints than other surfaces. Depending on the surface material, a local high school track may provide a consistent and more cushioned surface than pavement. Regardless of where you walk, invest in a good pair of walking shoes that will support and cushion your feet, ankles, and knees.

When you start walking, always do less than you think you should. If you think you can walk for ten minutes, start with seven minutes. If you think you can walk for twenty minutes, start with fifteen minutes. This will decrease the likelihood of triggering any additional symptoms. Do not attempt a walking program if you have any type of injury or disease exacerbated by walking.

Clinical Findings

One study measured the benefits of high-intensity walking on a treadmill against low-intensity walking on a treadmill. Low-intensity walking yielded more positive results, while high-intensity walking produced greater pain and a higher drop-out rate.

Cycling

Cycling is another low-impact activity that builds strength and increases endurance while minimizing stress on your joints and muscles. I recommend starting with an indoor stationary bicycle set at a low resistance. One of the benefits of stationary bicycles is that you can easily adjust the resistance to a setting that feels comfortable for you. Choose a stationary bicycle on which you can sit upright rather than in a hunched-over position. There are also bikes that allow you to sit with your back supported (recumbent bikes). This will reduce any stress on your upper body that may occur if you are in an awkward or uncomfortable position. If you have problems with grip strength, you can use a stationary bicycle without handlebars. Electronic stationary bicycles have a variety of settings—from flatwork to intense hill climbs. When you are getting started, keep the setting at a constant resistance that mimics riding down a perfectly flat street. Also, set the seat height high enough or far enough back so that your leg is almost completely straight when it is at the bottom of the spin; this will reduce wear on your knees.

Yoga, Tai Chi, and Pilates

Many of my patients have discovered that they enjoy the physical and mental aspects of yoga, Pilates, tai chi, and other programs that offer a mind-body approach to physical fitness. Yoga and tai chi are rooted in Eastern philosophies that encourage focused breathing, balanced movement, and a quiet, relaxed mind. These activities promote flexibility, increased range of motion, core strength, and relaxation. Each of these activities is taught in a wide variety of formats and at multiple skill levels.

Prior to attending a class, be sure to consult with the instructor to determine whether the class is suitable for you.

The best introduction to any of these practices is through private lessons. An instructor can teach you how to perform different movements and stretches in a way that minimizes the risk of injury. If private lessons are not affordable, try finding a class designed for older adults or for people with physical disabilities. These classes will generally offer a gentle introduction to the activity and teach various modifications of different poses. If you do join a class, don't compare yourself to others or try any position or repetition that seems likely to cause you increased pain. Classes range from forty-five to seventy-five minutes in length, which may be a long time for you to participate in any activity. Don't feel like you have to stay for the whole class. Most instructors will encourage you to take resting poses if you become tired and need a break, or you may decide to do only part of the class until you feel ready to do more. Another advantage of doing these activities is having the opportunity to practice them at home with the help of an instructional video. I recommend spending time in a class that offers some individualized instruction prior to working with these programs at home. In a class, you can always ask questions or get clarification. Once you get a feel for the activity, ask your instructor for video recommendations.

Yoga

Far more than a glorified stretching class, yoga originated in ancient India as a spiritual path to enlightenment through the union of the spiritual and physical self. Increasingly popular as a form of exercise in the United States, many yoga classes remain true to the mind-body component of this ancient tradition. Yoga helps tame the fight-or-flight response, as it calms the mind through focused breathing and a flowing sequence of body postures. You must be extremely careful not to overstretch while practicing yoga. There are many kinds of yoga. Iyengar and hatha are two styles that offer a gentle introduction to yoga. Proper form is critical when it comes to yoga, and finding an instructor who is knowledgeable enough and skilled enough to modify stretches and poses is essential for most people with fibromyalgia to avoid injury.

Clinical Findings

People who practice yoga don't need research to tell them just how great it is for the body and mind. Nevertheless, researchers are stumbling over each other to study how yoga might help everyone from cancer survivors to asthma sufferers.

A 2005 study enrolled twenty-four emotionally distressed women in a three-month yoga program. The women experienced significant improvement in perceived stress, anxiety, well-being, vigor, fatigue, and depression. Participants suffering from headache or back pain reported significant relief as well.

Tai Chi

Tai chi is a Chinese martial art dating back to the sixth century. Like yoga, the movements in tai chi have spiritual and philosophical origins. Tai chi instructors teach a sequence of flowing movements as a meditative exercise for the body and mind. Tai chi may be ideal for fibromyalgia patients, as its slow sequence of movements gradually increases muscle strength and improves flexibility. Tai chi also improves balance, coordination, and alignment. The meditative qualities of tai chi promote relaxation and ease stress.

Clinical Findings

Researchers studied the benefits of tai chi for fibromyalgia patients who took classes twice a week for six weeks. Results indicated improvement in symptom management and health-related quality of life. Other studies have found that tai chi lowers blood pressure, reduces the risk of falling for the elderly, and improves the overall quality of life for people with chronically disabling conditions, such as multiple sclerosis.

Pilates

Pilates is the new kid on the block when compared with the ancient traditions of yoga and tai chi. Developed by the German-born Joseph Pilates in the early 1900s, Pilates is a gentle and effective way to strengthen and stretch all the muscles in your body. Pilates uses the weight of the body itself to develop lean and flexible muscles through a series of repetitive movements. Pilates works to strengthen the body's core muscles, improving posture and alignment. Although Pilates is relatively new, many of its techniques are derived from yoga. Again, technique is everything, and finding the right instructor or class is essential. No formal research has been conducted on the benefits of Pilates for fibromyalgia patients. In the end, all that matters is whether a specific type of exercise benefits you.

Stretching Guidelines

- Warm up your muscles before stretching. Although most people think they should stretch before they exercise, stretching cold muscles is more likely to result in muscle damage. You can warm up your muscles by taking a hot bath or by slowly starting your aerobic activity and then taking a break to stretch.
- Perform stretching shortly after starting your exercise and again when you're through exercising.
- Always stretch slowly and carefully. Stretch until you reach the point of resistance but not the point of pain. It is also effective to move a body part slowly through a range of motion until a stretch is felt, and gently repeat that motion for thirty to sixty seconds.
- Try to hold each stretch for thirty seconds. If it is painful, back off a little and try it again. Don't hesitate to stretch for shorter periods if thirty seconds is too long for you to hold a position, and don't ever try to push through pain with stretches.

Physical Activity Wish List

Fibromyalgia can make every aspect of life extremely difficult. It's hard to track progress because as you improve, it's easy to forget just how bad things were even a month ago. Setting goals will help you measure any progress you make, no matter how small. List any physical activities you can no longer do because of fibromyalgia. These can include daily chores, sports, social gatherings, work, etc. List them in three groups, depending on how close you are to obtaining them.

After six weeks of exercise, take a look at this list and see if you have met any of your goals. Continue to measure your progress against this goal sheet. Write down the date next to a goal when you can take it off your wish list and add it back into your life.

Short-Term Activity Goals (e.g.: make the bed, take the dog for a walk, prepare dinner)

Midrange Activity Goals (e.g.: have energy all day, work in the garden, play with the kids)

Long-Range Activity Goals (e.g.: resume work full-time, run a 5K race)

Tracking Your Progress

Here are some ideas for charting your progress. Remember, everybody is different, and what may be easy for you may be difficult for someone else, and vice versa. These are by no means the only things you can keep track of, but these are commonly mentioned by my patients. I've organized the list in order of difficulty. This is only a guide. Remember that the relative difficulty of tasks may be much different from person to person. Take what is useful for you from the list in terms of *your* level, and see how you progress over time.

Light stretches

Walk 5–10 min. or one to two city blocks

Water plants

Lift gallon of milk from fridge

Make bed

Climb stairs < 8 stairs

Prepare and cook one meal

Work on computer 30–60 min.

Light cleaning

Light gardening > 45 min.

Mop the floor < 20 min.

Climb multiple flights of stairs > 2

Wash and clean car

Vacuum house

Walk 20–30 min.

Grocery store trip

Exercise 2 to 3 times/week, low intensity

Shopping > 2 hrs.

Work on computer > 2–3 hrs.

Exercise 2 times/week, moderate intensity (heart rate > 60% of target heart rate)

Weed garden > 60 min.

Rake leaves > 30 min.

Walk > 60 min.

Mow lawn

Ride bike on flat surfaces > 60 min.

Hike on even surfaces > 45 min.

Clean house 1 time/week

Exercise 3 to 4 times/week, moderate intensity (heart rate > 60% of target heart rate)

Shovel snow > 45 min.

In a Nutshell . . .

- If you have fibromyalgia, exercise may seem out of the question because of your pain and fatigue. However, a carefully designed exercise program can help you more than it hurts.
- The gradual reduction of daily activities associated with fibromyalgia contributes to muscle knots, muscle tension, loss of flexibility, and a decreased range of motion. As your muscles become deconditioned, daily activities will take more energy and cause more fatigue.
- Movement is medicine for your muscles. You need to find the right type and amount for your body.
- A successful exercise program is not measured in distance, repetitions, or speed. Your success with exercise will be measured by improvements in your energy and your ability to enjoy daily activities.
- Always start an exercise program slowly! Do less than you think you can. There's no such thing as a "good" sore if you have fibromyalgia.
- High-intensity aerobic exercise has no benefits over low-intensity aerobic exercise for people with fibromyalgia. Water aerobics and swimming are the best options for improving strength, flexibility, and endurance without increasing pain. Walking and cycling are also good options. Yoga, tai chi, and Pilates are recommended for gentle stretching and increasing core strength.
- Choose an exercise you enjoy, and make a commitment to yourself to stick with it.
- Consult with a physician or physical therapist if you have any concerns about your ability to exercise without exacerbating your symptoms.

CHAPTER 10

A New Type of Drug for Fibromyalgia

Most of the chapters in part 2 of this book involve making lifestyle changes that serve to either reverse your fibromyalgia triggers or alleviate your symptoms. So far, these lifestyle changes have included recommendations on how to improve sleep, reduce stress, make key dietary changes, and improve your physical fitness. Each of these lifestyle changes will not only speed you along the road to recovery but will help you maintain a healthy, active lifestyle long after you have recovered from fibromyalgia. This chapter discusses the role of medication in treating fibromyalgia. Although medication plays an important role in helping many people recover, it is more often than not a short-term solution rather than a long-term necessity. In fact, a 2004 article published in the *Journal of the American Medical Association* found that exercise, cognitive-behavioral therapy (as described in chapter 7), and patient education were equally effective or more effective than most of the medications described in this chapter. Most of the medications discussed in this chapter are designed to help you feel good enough to follow the other components of the program described in part 2 of this book. Of course, if you feel that you can implement the lifestyle changes without the help of medications, you should start there. However, if you feel overwhelmed by pain and fatigue, you may benefit from working with your doctor to determine whether some of the medications described in this chapter are right for you. Once you are able to start working on your fibromyalgia triggers, you will become less and less dependent on medication to control your symptoms. Eventually, you should even be able to stop taking medication as you resolve your fibromyalgia triggers and begin to recover.

Most doctors prescribe medications to fibromyalgia patients in an attempt to help with their diverse array of symptoms. Prescribing medication for people with fibromyalgia has always been a tricky business. People are in pain, and doctors want to help. They prescribe a variety of medications that usually help people in pain, but as you know, fibromyalgia is not your typical kind of pain. Throw into the mix the fact that fibromyalgia symptoms vary on a day-to-day basis, and it's hard to know whether the medications are actually helping. Without a true understanding of how fibromyalgia works, this approach is often hit or miss. Whenever I meet a new patient, I take a close look at his or her medication list. Most people are taking several different drugs on a daily basis in a desperate attempt to control their symptoms. In most of these cases, people are taking far more medications than is really necessary, and many times they're not even taking the medications that would be most likely to provide relief.

One of the most important pieces of information that we now have in treating fibromyalgia is that the triggers vary from individual to individual. Finding the right medication involves not only determining that someone has fibromyalgia but also targeting how he or she developed fibromyalgia in the first place and identifying the person's current triggers. Without a special emphasis on the fibromyalgia triggers for a particular patient, prescribing medication is akin to treating any infection, regardless of whether it is due to stepping on a rusty nail or tuberculosis, with the exact same medication. Fibromyalgia must be thought of as a syndrome with many different triggers. Once you determine your particular triggers, you can work with your healthcare provider to determine the appropriate medications for you.

There are essentially three reasons I prescribe medications to my fibromyalgia patients. I am either trying to resolve underlying medical problems, attempting to help alleviate fibromyalgia symptoms, or in severe cases, striving to help stimulate dopamine production. In this chapter, I'll help you better understand the medications currently being used to help alleviate fibromyalgia symptoms and decide whether these medications might be appropriate in your situation. If you are currently taking a lot of medications, as most fibromyalgia patients are, there's a good chance you will be able to stop taking medications that are not actually helping. In this chapter, I'll also discuss the tremendous success I've had with the dopamine agonists: a revolutionary approach to treating fibromyalgia with medications that help replace your body's depleted dopamine. These are the same medications, described in part 1 of this book, that provided a key link in understanding the science behind fibromyalgia. Unlike other drugs used to provide some relief from the symptoms of fibromyalgia, these drugs actually help eliminate symptoms by replacing dopamine. By the end of this chapter, you should be able to work intelligently with your doctor to determine which medications are the most likely to help you feel better as you begin other aspects of your recovery plan. Once you have successfully followed the rest of the program described in part 2 of this book, you will find that you no longer need any medications that were prescribed for the short-term relief of symptoms.

Determining the Role of Medication in a Patient's Recovery Plan

In order for me to effectively prescribe medications for a fibromyalgia patient, it is essential that I have a good understanding of my patient's case history. A patient's case history helps me determine whether there are any underlying medical issues that could be causing pain, lets me know what other medications have been tried in the past and whether they provided any relief, and helps me decide whether medication might assist this patient as he or she starts a recovery plan. The case history you created in chapter 5 will be extremely important in helping you work with a doctor to determine whether specific medications might provide relief from underlying medical problems or offer help with fibromyalgia symptoms in the short term.

Once I diagnose a patient with fibromyalgia, I work with the patient and review the case history to determine the initial steps of his or her recovery plan. If I determine that a portion of the person's suffering stems from an underlying medical condition that can be helped through medication, I will prescribe the appropriate medication. Appropriate medications are essential for treating underlying medical conditions that may trigger or contribute to fibromyalgia. If a doctor assumes that all of a patient's symptoms are from fibromyalgia, it will be impossible to effectively treat underlying conditions. For example, if a patient also suffers from lupus or rheumatoid arthritis, I can prescribe medications to reduce symptoms caused by those particular problems. If some of a patient's fatigue stems from a thyroid problem, the right dose of thyroid hormone can provide a big boost to a patient's energy level. If someone has a bad case of tendonitis, a round of anti-inflammatory medication may reduce a great deal of pain. By determining any underlying medical conditions for each individual patient, I can move medication from the hit-or-miss category into the effective category. Of course, in some cases, the underlying medical condition may require a different intervention, such as surgery or physical therapy.

After I address underlying physical and medical causes, I then work with the patient to determine whether medication should play a role in the rest of the recovery plan. The most effective avenue of treatment is always chosen using a team approach between patient and physician. Common sense generally dictates the degree to which medication should play a role in the person's recovery. For example, if we discover that a person suffers from undiagnosed sleep apnea, I would treat this condition before prescribing any medication for fibromyalgia symptoms. The person's fibromyalgia could very well resolve as soon as the sleep apnea is improved. I almost always find that once I have explained how fibromyalgia actually works, the treatment path becomes very clear.

Keep in mind that there are no medications that have been approved by the Food and Drug Administration (FDA) for the express purpose of treating fibromyalgia. Many of the drugs currently prescribed to help fibromyalgia patients are prescribed to treat a specific symptom, such as depression or pain. In these cases, the doctor is prescribing a drug that has been approved to treat depression or pain rather than a drug that has been approved to treat fibromyalgia. Whenever a doctor prescribes a medication to treat fibromyalgia, the medication is being prescribed "off label." An off-label use simply means that the doctor is prescribing a drug to treat a condition other than the conditions approved by the FDA and listed on the drug's labeling. Off-label prescriptions are legal. The off-label use of prescription medications for fibromyalgia is quite common, as there are several medications that have shown promising results in their ability to help fibromyalgia patients feel better. Many of these treatments are likely to remain off label, because in order to gain FDA approval, a drug maker must do extensive testing of medications on that particular condition. The approval process is rigorous, testing both safety and efficacy. This is virtually impossible to do for a condition without a known cause, which is how most of the world still views fibromyalgia. As a result, most treatments are considered experimental in nature, and the results vary from patient to patient.

If you do elect to try any of the medications described below as part of your recovery plan, you should do so in conjunction with the lifestyle changes described in this part of the book. In order to determine whether a particular medication is helping you, keep track of how much you take and how it makes you feel in your Progress Journal. You can track your medications on a daily or weekly basis. The following sample chart illustrates one way to track your medications:

Date	Jan. 6–Jan. 12	Jan. 13–Jan. 19
Medication	Mirapex	Mirapex
Dose	.25 mg	.375 mg
Symptom Relief?	Maybe some—hard to really tell yet	Not feeling so tired during the day; thinking more clearly
Side Effects?	Somewhat sick to my stomach. Makes me sleepy.	Still makes me sick to my stomach, but getting better. Only happens in the evening.

The Dopamine Drugs

The dopamine drugs are an exciting new category of fibromyalgia medications. Until now, doctors only knew to prescribe medications that might provide relief from the many symptoms of fibromyalgia. Now that we understand how fibromyalgia actually works, it is possible to prescribe medications that get at the heart of fibromyalgia and boost dopamine levels. As you now understand, depleted dopamine causes most of your painful symptoms. Mirapex (pramipexole) and Requip (ropinirole) are medications typically prescribed for Parkinson's disease patients who suffer from dopamine depletion in a different part of the brain. When given to fibromyalgia patients, these medications are remarkably effective at relieving or eliminating fibromyalgia pain, because they work by replacing dopamine, allowing your autonomic nervous system to once again filter unwanted sensations.

In August 2005, Dr. Andrew Holman, the acknowledged pioneer in the field of dopamine agonists and fibromyalgia, published the results of a major placebo-controlled trial testing Mirapex in the treatment of fibromyalgia. Dr. Holman proved that Mirapex, when compared with a placebo, was very helpful in treating the symptoms of fibromyalgia. The patients taking Mirapex had less pain, functioned better, and had more energy than those taking the placebo. Nearly all of the participants in the study improved on some measure. Almost half of the participants taking Mirapex had a greater than 50 percent reduction in their pain after just fourteen weeks! The main side effects included weight loss, anxiety, diarrhea, and morning tiredness.

I first began using Mirapex with a few of my fibromyalgia patients in 2001. The patients I treated with Mirapex soon started to show dramatic improvements. They started thinking more clearly and sleeping better. Their energy level improved, and their painful sensations started to resolve. In short, patients who could take this drug started to feel as though they'd gotten their lives back. Needless to say, with these encouraging results, I started using Mirapex with even more of my patients. Virtually all of those who were able to take the medication got significantly better. For people who couldn't tolerate Mirapex, I started them on Requip. Although not always as effective, Requip has fewer side effects.

For many people, these drugs seem like a cure for fibromyalgia. However, you have to keep in mind that although these drugs correct the most important imbalance in fibromyalgia and therefore eliminate most of the symptoms, they do not actually cure fibromyalgia. Fibromyalgia is caused by a prolonged activation of the fight-or-flight response, which results in an imbalance of all the body's stress hormones and many other chemicals and neurotransmitters. If the only thing keeping you trapped in the fibromyalgia cycle is the pain and exhaustion of fibromyalgia, then these drugs can break the cycle of pain and essentially cure you. However, as I discussed earlier, most people have other fibromyalgia triggers that must also be resolved before they are truly cured of fibromyalgia. Therefore, I always prescribe these drugs as one step of many along the road to recovery. Let's take a look at how these drugs typically help people recover from fibromyalgia.

First of all, patients must start taking these medications at very low doses. It can take several months of slowly increasing the dosage before a patient reaches the optimal dose. During this time, the patient will begin to sleep better and think more clearly. As the patient's pain starts to recede, he or she will also experience a lessening of the fight-or-flight response. Once the patient begins to feel better, work can begin on his or her specific fibromyalgia triggers as the patient implements all the elements of the recovery plan. This may involve addressing psychological issues or treating underlying medical causes. After the patient successfully achieves each step of the recovery plan, he or she can slowly start to reduce the use of these drugs. This could take as little as six months or as long as several years, depending on the person's particular triggers. True recovery takes place when a patient is able to discontinue the dopamine drugs and none of the symptoms return.

Side Effects

If you do decide to try Mirapex or Requip, you have to approach this protocol knowing full well that there's a good chance you won't be one of the lucky ones able to easily tolerate these drugs. If you're not able to take these drugs, don't panic. There are some additional pharmaceutical options for relieving your symptoms, which I will discuss later in this chapter.

In my experience, Mirapex and Requip are both reasonably safe if used very carefully. No damaging effects have been observed in the liver, kidneys, or any other organ tissues. However, some people find the side effects hard to tolerate. Nearly 80 percent of my patients experience some nausea. In most cases, it is mild and can be treated. Often, the nausea simply goes away with time. There's no disputing that nausea as a side effect is unpleasant, but it can generally be treated effectively with ginger or medications, such as Phenergan (promethazine) Compazine (prochlorperazine), and Zofran (ondansetron). In addition, acid blockers such as Prilosec (omeprazole), Pepto Bismol (bismuth), or Pepcid AC (famotidine) can be quite helpful. For even more assistance, you may want to ask your doctor about Nexium (esomeprazole) or Prevacid (lansoprazole).

People who take these medications can grow sleepy or confused, so caution must always be exercised when driving. According to the *Physician's Desk Reference,* there have been reports of automobile accidents associated with patients who are using either Mirapex or Requip to treat Parkinson's disease. The key difference to bear in mind is that Parkinson's patients are advised to take the medications around the clock, whereas for fibromyalgia patients, the medications should only be used just before bedtime, so they cause sleepiness at the very moment you want to go to sleep. In my own medical practice, I've only had to stop the medications for three patients due to daytime sleepiness. You should never drive if you experience daytime sleepiness associated with these medications.

Some patients actually have too much energy once they are on these medications. In my experience, patients who are anxious and tend toward very high adrenaline levels are more likely to experience this effect. For people who experience increased energy with these drugs, it may be difficult to sleep. In those instances—if I feel I can trust them not to drive—I have them take their medications in the morning. As the dose gets increased and the patients become sleepy during the day, I ask them to shift over to the more common practice of taking their medications just before bedtime.

One troubling side effect is that for people with bipolar disorder, these drugs can exacerbate the mania. In a way, this makes sense, as dopamine is essentially a stimulant. When a person becomes unusually talkative or starts to exhibit far too much energy, it may indicate the onset of a manic episode. When treating bipolar patients, I only prescribe these medications as part of a program developed in conjunction with the patients' psychiatrists, and even then, only if provisions have been made for closely monitoring the patients.

For patients who also have restless legs syndrome (RLS), the restless jerking may worsen before it gets better. In most cases, this will normalize over time. But there are rare instances in which it continues to get worse and worse. In those cases, the medications will have to be stopped. This phenomenon is called amplification and is well known among physicians who regularly treat people with RLS. Occasionally, the amplification can be overcome with the help of such drugs as Ativan (lorazepam), Xanax (alprazolam), and Klonopin (clonazepam), which are the same drugs I use to lower patients' adrenaline level enough so they can sleep at night. I also often use these same medications in combination with Mirapex and/or Requip.

One other recent side effect reported with the use of Mirapex in treating Parkinson's disease is excessive gambling or other compulsive behaviors such as excessive spending. Although not common, I discuss this with all my patients and their spouses or families and ask that they be involved, watching for these potentially destructive behaviors. Patients who develop these behaviors usually have to decrease or stop the medication. Other less likely side effects include anxiety, tremors, worsening sleep, exceptionally vivid dreams, confusion, light-headedness, hair thinning, excitation, fluid retention, tremulousness, and, rarely, hallucinations. Excitation or anxiety can certainly worsen, as dopamine is a stimulant. Besides worsening sleep and possibly causing undesirable behaviors, patients describe this as being revved up or feel like their bodies are buzzing. At times, this can be overcome with medications such as Buspar (buspirone) or Paxil (paroxetine). I feel the best way to deal with this scenario is to lower the dose until the sensations are tolerable while the patients work on controlling the fight-or-flight response. Even low doses can be helpful if taken while the patients work on their fibromyalgia triggers.

Some people suffer from tremors that can get worse with these medications. The most common tremor condition is called benign essential tremor. This usually comes on as people age and involves an uncontrollable shaking. This generally involves the hand, but it can also involve the head or voice. Essential tremor worsens when the body is stimulated, such as during an infection or after drinking caffeine. This side effect is reversible and can also be improved by lowering the dose.

I have had to stop these medications in several patients who were having exceptionally vivid dreams. This can happen with any drug that affects the central nervous system (CNS), including over-the-counter medications such as melatonin. This is a rare side effect that may resolve in a week or two. If not, you should lower the dose gradually and eventually stop the medications.

Confusion is also possible with any medications that affect the CNS. This is much more likely to occur if you are older than fifty or are taking other medications that affect the brain, such as antidepressants or antianxiety medications. The confusion is similar to the fibro fog I describe earlier in the book. If you find yourself forgetting what you were talking about or unable to remember where you put things, the medications may be to blame. If the confusion does not resolve after a few weeks or becomes a problem, these medications may not be right for you.

Some people experience light-headedness on these medications. My patients report feeling dizzy or as if they are about to faint whenever they stand up or change positions quickly. This usually happens because the medications decrease your body's ability to raise blood pressure quickly when you change positions. This is much more likely to happen if you are over sixty or already have problems with light-headedness or low blood pressure. If this continues for more than a few days, the medication dosage must be lowered or stopped.

Fluid retention, or edema, can happen with either drug, but it is more common with Mirapex. Since patients with fibromyalgia are much more likely to notice discomfort from fluid retention, this is a somewhat frequent side effect, occurring in approximately 10 percent of patients. It can be treated by lowering the dose or adding a diuretic (a water pill). This may also be a cause of a minor weight gain. However, most patients lose weight with these medications.

Hallucinations are a rare side effect that usually occurs at night. In the few patients with this side effect, all were taking another medication that affected the CNS, such as Ambien (zolpidem), a prescription sleep medication. This side effect can be treated by lowering the dose and/or stopping the other medications.

Many of the above side effects will be more likely to occur if you have other medical conditions or are taking certain medications. For example, if you have irritable bowel syndrome or heartburn, nausea and stomach upset are much more likely to occur. If you are over sixty years old, the gastrointestinal side effects are usually less tolerable. In addition, older patients are more likely to experience sleepiness during the day, become confused, and retain fluid. Patients with untreated sleep apnea tend to have more nausea with these medications. As I already mentioned, anxiety can be worsened by these medications. Some patients with depression become more depressed, but this is rare. Most become less depressed as their symptoms improve. If you already suffer from dementia, these medications will likely worsen your thinking and should only be used under the strictest supervision.

Certain medications can also make it less likely that you will tolerate the dopamine agonists. Stimulants, such as Adipex (phentermine), a prescription diet medication, or Adderall (amphetamines), a prescription stimulant for narcolepsy, can combine with dopamine to worsen anxiety. I usually don't combine the dopamine agonists with these powerful stimulants, but low doses of each may be tolerated. Other medications such as Prozac, a stimulating antidepressant, may worsen anxiety if combined with a dopamine agonist. As you review your medications with your physician, look out for any additive effects caused by other medications if you notice increased anxiety with the dopamine medications.

This additive effect is true of other medications. If you are taking sleep aids, you may find that once combined with a dopamine agonist, you are much sleepier at night and have trouble waking up in the morning. If this happens or if you experience a "hangover," you may be able to lower the dose of the sleep aid. This decision, as with all medication decisions, must be discussed with your prescribing physician. Never make these vital decisions on your own.

Side effects are more likely to occur if you take these medications in combination with other medications with similar side effects. If you are taking medications that can cause nausea, fluid retention, confusion, or light-headedness, consider asking your physician which medications might be implicated if you notice these side effects. The list of medications with these possible side effects is endless. This makes prescribing these medications and dealing with the side effects a team effort between patient and physician.

In my experience, I've found that the people least likely to tolerate these medications are those who already have a history of stomach problems and have already had to stop taking other medications due to stomach problems or nausea. Also, if you are over sixty, suffer from untreated sleep apnea, or have certain forms of neck arthritis, the chances are greater that you may have difficulties with these medications.

Dosage

In the paragraphs that follow, I'll summarize what I've learned from my experience so that both you and your primary care physician will have a better idea of what to expect. Keep in mind that the following protocol is an off-label therapy that has not been approved by the FDA. Although many doctors have been willing to try this therapy with their patients, yours may hesitate. In a society as litigious as ours, healthcare providers can be quite reluctant to get involved with off-label therapies. That's understandable, but unfortunately it's the patients who suffer as a result. A model consent form has been included at the end of this book. This form helps safeguard your physician from a lawsuit in the event that you should experience any unforeseeable side effects from these drugs. You may need to use it—or one like it—to alleviate any fear your primary care physician may have about prescribing you a dopamine agonist. Remember that these drugs are still very new in the treatment of fibromyalgia. Caution must still be exercised throughout your treatment, as physicians and researchers may discover new side effects as more and more people use the drugs.

You also may want to check with your pharmacist to see if you have adequate insurance coverage. These drugs can be expensive but are usually covered by most major insurers. Requip is approved for the treatment of RLS, which most patients with fibromyalgia also suffer from. This can help get the medication covered by some insurers. Some of my patients decide to pay for the medications themselves if they don't have adequate insurance. Although expensive, they may only be needed for several months if other triggers are adequately addressed.

I always start by prescribing Mirapex, since it is the more potent of the two drugs. In the event that a patient cannot tolerate Mirapex, I switch him or her to Requip. The optimal dose of Mirapex for eliminating most symptoms is 4.5 mg. At doses higher than this, side effects increase, and fewer benefits are seen. I typically start patients with an initial dose of just 0.125 mg per day, taken just before bedtime. I'll then step up the daily dosage by 0.125 mg with each passing week while I monitor how the patient responds, up to 0.375 mg per night. This slow increase is vital to the body's ability to get accustomed to this medication. Even somewhat severe side effects can improve with time, even as the patient continues to slowly increase the dosage. It's very important for patients to maintain a consistent regimen, since they can experience extreme nausea should they take a medication break. If they end up skipping a few days, they may need to rebuild the dosage slowly again, albeit not quite as slowly as the first time.

If the patient can tolerate the medication, I'll then launch into the full protocol—0.5 mg tablets prescribed for nightly usage. Thereafter, I step up the daily dosage by another 0.25 mg with each passing week until patients are taking 2 mg per night. If patients are doing well at 2 mg per night after 8 weeks, I begin increasing the dose in 0.75 mg increments every two weeks until patients reach the ideal dose of 4.5 mg per night.

In the event a patient is unable to take Mirapex, I start him or her on Requip. I start patients with 0.25 mg and then increase the dosage by 0.25 mg each week to .75 mg. If this is tolerated, the patients can then take 1 mg each night, increasing to a nightly maximum of 12 to 15 mg over a like number of weeks. In general, patients who find they can't tolerate Mirapex at all still have a reasonable chance of being able to handle Requip.

In my view, "tolerating the medication" means having few or no side effects, or at least side effects that you can live with. And that's important—not simply because of comfort, but also because interrupted sleep and severe nausea are unlikely to lower your fight-or-flight response activity. You should definitely stop the medications if you experience any major side effects or find that the side effects aren't resolving promptly.

If necessary, this stepwise increase in dosage can be slowed. Also, for those who manage to make headway against fibromyalgia at lower doses, there's really no reason to step up the dosage. You can always do that later, should progress slow or plateau at any point. Also, should it turn out that the maximum tolerated dose of Mirapex isn't quite enough to rein in your symptoms, you can consider supplementing it with Requip. Generally, in such instances, I add Requip at .25 mg, build to 1 mg, and then step up the protocol by 1 mg per week. By and large, the Requip dose needs to be three times larger than the Mirapex dose to net the same effect. For example, if you can only tolerate 1.5 mg of Mirapex a day—instead of the optimal 4.5 mg—then you should probably aim to replace the missing 3 mg with 9 mg of Requip. It will take you at least nine weeks to reach that level.

These medications should not be stopped abruptly once they are being taken at high doses. It is possible that a rare side effect similar to neuroleptic malignant syndrome (NMS), which can bring on fever, confusion, low blood pressure, and shortness of breath, could occur. Patients should always be weaned off these medications over a few days to a week. Although there are no recorded instances of NMS associated with Mirapex or Requip discontinuation, it has been noted with other drugs from the same pharmacological family. Although extremely rare, your healthcare provider should explain this syndrome and the need to wean off these medications somewhat slowly. Drug interactions should also be reviewed with your health-care provider and pharmacist.

If you can tolerate these medications, the pattern of recovery usually goes like this. First, you'll notice that your body's restless jerking will start to subside. Then, you'll find that your sleep improves and your energy increases. After that, you can expect your confusion to clear up. And then, once you're up to the higher doses, you'll find that your sensations aren't quite so amplified and that your pain has subsided. Although this is the general order in which improvements occur, there is no set time frame for improvements. Patients with mild to moderate fibromyalgia may notice significant improvement, including pain relief, within the first few weeks. People with more severe fibromyalgia may not notice similar improvements until they have reached the highest doses of Mirapex or Requip, as they are suffering from more severe dopamine depletion. However, once you achieve the optimal dose for your body, you will improve. In fact, the improvements that can be realized with Mirapex and Requip are so palpable that even those patients who can't tolerate the drugs well at higher doses may choose to stay on a low, more tolerable dose of the medication to gain some partial relief from the miseries of fibromyalgia.

It's possible that you might follow the off-label protocol and yet realize little, if any, progress. In that event, consider the possibility that your pain may be due to something else, such as lupus or osteoarthritis. The dopamine drugs will only provide relief if it's fibromyalgia you're suffering from. Keep in mind that the dopamine agonists are so uniformly effective in the fight against fibromyalgia that you can be reasonably certain that something else is wrong if the higher doses of Mirapex or Requip fail to reduce your discomfort.

There are cases, such as when a patient has sleep apnea, when the advantages afforded by the dopamine agonists may be minimal. If your body thinks it's dying every night (due to suffocation from sleep apnea), there isn't any drug strong enough to control the corresponding stress response you have night after night. The significance of this was brought home to me when several patients of mine who didn't respond favorably to Mirapex were eventually found to have sleep apnea. In addition, certain forms of neck arthritis can raise your adrenaline level, thus undercutting the benefits of Mirapex therapy in much the same way sleep apnea does. In the 1990s, a specific surgical procedure to relieve this pressure at the base of the brain was developed—one of the more drastic treatments tried for fibromyalgia. This procedure can provide some benefit whenever neck arthritis is found to be actively contributing to the fibromyalgia cycle.

Fortunately, Mirapex can be combined with most other medications. In addition, you may be surprised to find that once your adrenaline level has normalized, all your other medications start to work better. That's particularly true for those medications intended to help you relax or sleep. The same drugs that failed to help you sleep at one time may suddenly become much too strong for you once you've started to rebuild your dopamine stores. You and your primary healthcare provider may want to decrease or stop some other medications. For example, it may be that you slipped into a depression over time due to the pain you were in. But now that your pain has greatly diminished, you may find you no longer need an antidepressant. The same goes for any pain or sleep medications you may be taking.

Luckily, there are only a few drug interactions noted with the dopamine medications. A drug interaction is much more serious than both drugs working together to cause more nausea. A true drug interaction means that one drug you are taking greatly amplifies or reduces the effect of another drug through binding or blocking a receptor in your body for that drug. In general, drugs that interact in this way should not be taken together or should be taken at greatly reduced doses. Mirapex has only one major drug interaction—with the medication Tagamet (cimetidine), an acid blocker used to treat acid reflux. Only small doses of Mirapex should be used if you are taking Tagamet. However, there are many drugs similar to Tagamet that can easily be substituted. (Tagamet interacts with many medications.)

Requip should not be combined with the antibiotic Cipro (ciprofloxacin) due to the potential for a serious drug interaction. There are some other drugs that should not be taken with Requip due to the potential for minor interactions. Review any medications you are currently taking with your prescribing physician and your pharmacist before you start taking Requip. They can advise you if any of your medications might interact poorly with Requip.

Once you resolve your fibromyalgia triggers, you should continue to take Mirapex or Requip for another six to eight months to ensure that your body has a chance to fully replenish its supply of dopamine. In my experience, the medications are usually necessary until you begin to change the way the fight-or-flight response is used. Once you have your fight-or-flight response under control, these drugs can usually be safely lowered and eventually stopped. If the triggers persist, the drugs are usually still necessary. Ask yourself, "What triggers are activating my fight-or-flight response?" If you have a fibromyalgia trigger that cannot be adequately resolved, you may have to remain on these medications. However, don't use these medications as an excuse to avoid resolving your fibromyalgia triggers. We still don't know if they will retain their efficacy over the long term. If these medications lose their efficacy over time and you haven't resolved your fibromyalgia triggers, you'll be right back where you started.

Medications Commonly Used for Symptom Relief

Unlike Mirapex and Requip, the medications described in this section are only intended to improve your symptoms. Since they don't affect your dopamine levels, they won't eliminate symptoms to the extent that the dopamine drugs will. However, for people who can't or don't want to take Mirapex or Requip, many other medications can provide you with temporary relief of symptoms. Without this relief, some people will find it difficult to work on their triggers and focus on different aspects of recovery. Finding an easily tolerated medication that treats more than one trigger or symptom at a time can be a great help.

Medications that consistently provide short-term relief of fibromyalgia symptoms include those that treat depression or anxiety, relax muscles, or decrease nerve conduction. Most studies conducted on the efficacy of these drugs for fibromyalgia have been rather short, generally lasting six to twelve weeks, so the long-term efficacy is unknown. In some studies, drugs lost their effectiveness over a long period of time. However, this is not a problem for you, because you should only expect to take these drugs during the initial stages of recovery. Although this time frame is different for everyone, you should be able to discontinue medications expressly prescribed for symptomatic treatment within three months if you also make the other lifestyle changes of your recovery plan. If you find a drug that helps alleviate your symptoms and decide not to follow the other important elements of your recovery plan, there's a good chance that when the drug stops working, you'll be right back where you started. Be careful not to let the short-term benefits of these medications give you a false sense of security!

Antidepressants

Antidepressants are one of the most commonly prescribed medications for fibromyalgia. Medications for depression or anxiety are helpful for many patients. Even if you weren't anxious or depressed before you had fibromyalgia, the pain, stress, and sleep deprivation can cause depression or anxiety in virtually anyone. If so, these medications can help. Even if you are not depressed, some antidepressants have other beneficial effects, including improving sleep and reducing pain. There are three classes of antidepressants that can help alleviate fibromyalgia symptoms: tricyclic antidepressants, selective serotonin reuptake inhibitors (SSRIs), and serotonin/norepinephrine reuptake inhibitors (SNRIs). Let's take a look at some of the medications in these categories and discuss how they might help you.

Tricyclic Antidepressants

Tricyclic antidepressants have been available for over fifty years. These medications are generally taken at night and improve sleep, relax tense muscles, and heighten the effects of endorphins, which are natural painkillers in the body. Over the years, one of the most commonly prescribed medications for fibromyalgia patients has been Elavil (amitriptyline). When I went to medical school, I was taught to put every fibromyalgia patient on Elavil. Elavil not only treats depression but also induces sleep and is thought to slow nerve conduction. Clinical trials have demonstrated improvements in pain, sleep difficulties, fatigue, and tender-point scores with treatments of 25 to 50 mg of Elavil, taken at night. Your doctor may start you on a much lower dose and slowly increase it as needed. Weight gain and dry mouth are common side effects. There are other tricyclic antidepressants available. Most clinical trials of tricyclic antidepressants have lasted between six and twelve weeks. A longer trial reported that the improvements seen at six and twelve weeks were lost at twenty-six weeks. This is why I always recommend that patients take these medications in conjunction with making the lifestyle changes of their recovery plan. If, in the first six to twelve weeks of feeling better, you also improve your diet, work to reduce stress, and start sleeping better, you will be off to a great start in your overall recovery plan.

SSRIs

Prozac (fluoxetine) was the first of a new class of antidepressants that made treating depression with medication more popular. These drugs are called selective serotonin reuptake inhibitors (SSRIs). By selectively increasing serotonin levels, these drugs can be very effective for treating depression, fatigue, and other fibromyalgia symptoms. Many can also treat anxiety. This popular and expanding class of medications also includes Paxil (paroxetine) and Zoloft (sertraline). In a twelve-week placebo-controlled trial with Prozac, sixty women were treated with 10 to 80 mg of Prozac (dosage varied depending on the patient's needs, age, and tolerance). After twelve weeks, the women who took Prozac improved on a variety of measures, including pain and depression. A study that compared Zoloft with Elavil found that 50 mg of Zoloft was as effective as 25 mg of Elavil in reducing symptoms. Another study found that a combination of Prozac (20 mg) and Elavil

(25 mg) was more effective than either drug alone. Your physician can work with you to determine which medication or combination of medications might be most likely to help with your particular symptoms.

SNRIs

Cymbalta (duloxetine) is a new medication used for treating depression and pain. Cymbalta is a selective serotonin/norepinephrine reuptake inhibitor (SNRI) that acts on serotonin and norepinephrine, influencing both mood and pain. In addition to treating depression, Cymbalta slows nerve conduction in ways similar to Lyrica and Neurontin (described below). Many fibromyalgia patients who suffer from depression find Cymbalta very effective at alleviating their depression and reducing their pain. In addition, patients who don't suffer from depression may also find Cymbalta effective at reducing pain. In a 2005 placebo-controlled trial of Cymbalta, researchers found that 60 mg of Cymbalta, given once or twice a day, was effective at reducing pain in those with depression as well as those without depression.

Drugs That Slow Nerve Conduction

Drugs that slow nerve conduction, also known as anticonvulsant medications (antiseizure medications), can be very helpful for relieving pain, reducing anxiety, improving sleep, and reducing fatigue. Drugs traditionally used to stop seizures have also been used to treat chronic pain for many years because they work by slowing nerve conduction. In the case of fibromyalgia, these medications provide relief by slowing nerve conduction and preventing some pain impulses from reaching the brain. These drugs include Neurontin (gabapentin) and Lyrica (pregabalin).

Neurontin is an anticonvulsant approved for the treatment of seizures. However, it is commonly used off-label to treat many other conditions, including anxiety disorders, restless legs syndrome, chronic pain, and fibromyalgia. It is a relatively safe drug with fewer side effects than some antidepressants. One of the benefits for fibromyalgia patients is that Neurontin increases slow-wave sleep, a stage of sleep that is often disrupted in fibromyalgia patients. Side effects include sleepiness, dizziness, and problems with coordination. The National Institute of Arthritis and Musculoskeletal and Skin Diseases is currently funding a study to assess the efficacy of gabapentin (the generic form of Neurontin) in treating fibromyalgia symptoms.

This drug has recently been released in a more potent form, Lyrica (pregabalin). Lyrica is currently approved for the treatment of epilepsy and diabetic neuropathy. A 2005 placebo-controlled trial studied the effects of Lyrica on 529 fibromyalgia patients. This eight-week trial found that when given at 450 mg per day, it reduced pain by 50 percent for some patients. Patients who took dosages of 300 or 450 mg per day experienced significant improvements in sleep quality, fatigue, and other measures of change. The most commonly reported side effects were sleepiness and dizziness. It is likely that the drug's maker, Pfizer, will complete more studies and apply to the FDA for approval to use this drug in the treatment of fibromyalgia symptoms. In the meantime, doctors may prescribe this drug on an off-label basis.

Muscle Relaxants

Muscle relaxants help provide relief for some patients with fibromyalgia. Most people with fibromyalgia suffer from tensed muscles. Muscle relaxants help alleviate muscle contractions by decreasing the signal from the brain that makes the muscles contract. These drugs are also helpful for inducing sleep.

The most commonly prescribed muscle relaxant is Flexeril (cyclobenzaprine). Although generally prescribed as a muscle relaxant, Flexeril is structurally similar to the tricyclic antidepressants. In clinical trials, Flexeril has been effective at helping relieve symptoms in fibromyalgia patients when given at 10 to 40 mg per day. Because Flexeril makes people sleepy, I generally only prescribe it to be taken in the evenings. Muscle relaxants that can be safely used during the day are Skelaxin (metaxalone) and Norflex (orphenadrine). Many patients may use their muscle relaxants when they are having a particularly painful day. Your doctor will be able to help you decide if one of these medications is appropriate for your symptoms.

Commonly Prescribed and OTC Drugs That Don't Generally Work

The medications described below are commonly taken by fibromyalgia patients in an attempt to alleviate pain. Unfortunately, none of these medications is very effective, and you are probably causing more harm than good due to the side effects that result from the long-term use of some of them.

Nonsteroidal Anti-inflammatory Medications (NSAIDs)

This category of medications includes ibuprofen (Motrin, Advil) and naproxen sodium (Aleve, Anaprox). It's natural to think that these medications may have some effect, since they generally help relieve the aches and pains people commonly experience. However, these drugs work by reducing inflammation, and inflammation is not a side effect of fibromyalgia. If you find any relief from these medications, then you have another condition that is causing you pain in addition to fibromyalgia. A placebo-controlled study found no difference between ibuprofen and a placebo in the treatment of fibromyalgia. Naproxen sodium has failed to achieve notable improvements in a controlled trial. Ibuprofen can actually result in side effects that will make your fibromyalgia symptoms worse. These include ulcerations, abdominal pain, cramping, nausea, gastritis, and even serious gastrointestinal bleeding. Likewise, some of the more common side effects of naproxen sodium include abdominal pain, constipation, diarrhea, headaches, indigestion, and nausea.

Narcotics

The most controversial of medications prescribed for fibromyalgia are narcotics. Narcotics are the most potent pain medications available. They provide excellent relief in virtually all painful conditions—everything, that is, except fibromyalgia. Most patients will get relief when they first try these medicines. If you've ever taken Vicodin (hydrocodone), the commonly prescribed narcotic, you may still remember the first time you tried it. Usually it is the first thing that helped with your pain. You may have tried to clean your house for the first time in months. You may have even thought more clearly and felt more energy. Unfortunately, the relief narcotics provide is always short-lived. After a few weeks, they start to lose their potency. Before long, each pill seems to last only an hour or two. Instead of three pills a day, it now takes six to eight to get the same relief. Your healthcare provider may raise the potency of Vicodin or switch to something stronger, such as generic morphine. This may help for a few more weeks or maybe a month, but the relief usually fades with time. Not only are the higher doses of medications no better than that first Vicodin, but now there are more side effects. Constipation, confusion, and nausea, among others, may only be adding to your suffering. What is happening here?

Narcotics, in part, provide pain relief by increasing dopamine levels in the central nervous system. Narcotics only temporarily pump out more of this depleted dopamine, but after a few weeks, you are left with lower levels than ever. The narcotics will become less effective, but you might continue to take them or even be tempted to raise the dose in hopes of finding the relief they initially provided. I recommend that my patients who are currently taking narcotics maintain or even lower the dose while we add more effective medications and follow the other elements of their recovery plans. It should now be clear that there are far more effective options when it comes to treating fibromyalgia.

In a Nutshell . . .

- If your symptoms are severe, you may need to use medications for symptom relief before you can begin the other elements of your recovery plan.
- Medications for fibromyalgia are used to replace dopamine, treat underlying medical problems, and alleviate symptoms. Your symptoms and underlying medical conditions will dictate which medications are most effective for you.
- Mirapex and Requip are the first drugs that actually work to reverse the dopamine depletion that causes fibromyalgia.
- Only some people can tolerate the side effects, which include nausea and sleepiness. Those who can tolerate the side effects almost always start feeling better within weeks or a few months.
- Antidepressants, muscle relaxants, and drugs that slow nerve conduction are the most effective traditional drug therapies for fibromyalgia.
- Narcotics and nonsteroidal anti-inflammatory medications are not effective in the long-term treatment of fibromyalgia pain.

CHAPTER 11

Complementary Therapies

Frustrated by the mainstream medical community's lack of answers, fibromyalgia patients often look elsewhere for help. Complementary therapies are treatments that may help resolve underlying problems—such as an old injury or a strained muscle. They may also help alleviate some of your symptoms, including pain, helping you to feel better on a day-to-day basis. Many of these therapies will help you relax and give your body some much-deserved pampering. None of the therapies described below will cure fibromyalgia, but they may help speed the healing process and can play an important role in your recovery plan.

Unfortunately, once you are diagnosed with fibromyalgia, your doctor may mistakenly assume that the fibromyalgia itself is the only source of your pain. As we discussed, it can make matters worse if such treatable problems as stiff muscles, trigger points, or tendonitis are subsequently overlooked. It may be up to you to discuss the need for complementary therapies with your doctor. Remember—it's your body, and you know it better than you think you do. Don't dismiss all your pain as stemming from fibromyalgia. Fibromyalgia certainly makes your pain worse, but if you can reduce the number of true problem spots in your body, your pain will diminish as well.

Many of my patients have successfully used the therapies described below to either resolve underlying problems or find temporary relief from some of their symptoms. Please note that it is more useful to see a practitioner for a particular problem—such as a stiff neck or acutely painful shoulder—than to see someone just for fibromyalgia. The treatments described below will be most effective if they are addressing a specific physical problem that may be contributing to the pain you experience with fibromyalgia.

This chapter describes some of the most common and helpful treatments fibromyalgia patients generally turn to for symptom relief. They include the following:

- massage
- osteopathic manipulation
- chiropractic treatments
- physical therapy
- acupuncture
- trigger-point therapy

Where possible, I've described clinical findings that indicate whether these treatments are proven to provide relief. The most important thing is to choose treatments that make sense for *your* body and that *you* believe will help. Sometimes, your belief in a specific treatment is as important as the actual treatment in helping you feel better. It's important to remember that each case of fibromyalgia is unique and that what works for one person will not necessarily prove helpful for another. You should always base decisions about your treatment on your own particular symptoms. Although you can experiment with all of these treatments, I don't recommend mixing and matching in the beginning. It will be difficult to truly know what is effective if you try more than one type of treatment at a time. Also, it may put too much stress on your body to try more than one type of therapy in a short period of time. In order to determine whether a particular treatment is helping, make notes in your Progress Journal and track your symptoms as they increase or decrease following any particular treatment. Use the sample chart below to develop your own system for tracking any complementary therapies you try.

Date	June 17
Treatment	1 hr massage
How did it feel?	Found lots of sore, tender spots, but mostly felt good.
Later that day?	Shoulders feel more relaxed—feels great to take care of myself.
The next day?	Not a big difference, but muscles don't seem as tight.
Notes for next visit	Ask therapist to spend more time working on the tight areas in shoulders and upper back.

None of these therapies should hurt or cause you pain. In some cases, you may experience some residual or transient soreness in the days following a treatment. As long as the soreness is mild and temporary, there is no cause for concern. If you try a therapy and don't like it, then by all means try something else. But if something appeals to you, stick with it for a while and see what kind of results you can achieve. There is one exception: if you decide to have trigger-point therapy, you should schedule a massage on the same day, if at all possible. I'll explain why in the section on trigger-point therapy.

Massage

You already know that it feels good to have a friend or loved one massage your neck or rub a sore spot on your back. The lack of movement associated with fibromyalgia can increase muscle knots and muscle tension throughout the body. Stress also results in continually tensed muscles and the development of muscle knots. A professional massage therapist has extensive training in manipulating muscles and connective tissues to relieve tension, release knots, and restore range of motion. In addition to alleviating muscle tension, massage also improves circulation and may help release trigger points. Trigger points are taut bands of muscle that feel like hard, pea-size lumps under the skin. They can cause localized pain, but they also refer pain to other nearby areas.

Depending on your needs, you can either choose a full-body massage or you can ask the practitioner to focus on a particularly painful area of your body. Although a full-body massage can feel great, you may achieve more long-term benefits from a more focused massage. If you get a full-body, one-hour massage, the practitioner will not have time to really work on any problem areas. If you have truly tight spots, a practitioner will have to work slowly on one spot for a longer period of time in order to achieve any lasting result. With fibromyalgia patients in particular, a practitioner should always proceed slowly and gently. You can visit a massage therapist one to two days a week as long as you leave several days in between visits. You don't want to overwork your body. Results will vary depending on your particular needs, but you should start to notice a difference within two or three visits if massage is going to be beneficial for you.

Although massage has many benefits, deep-tissue massage may make your symptoms worse. If you decide to use massage as a treatment, choose a practitioner who is familiar with fibromyalgia. Ask the practitioner to start with gentle massage techniques that help relax the connective tissues and feel good to you. In the beginning, ask him or her to avoid working too deeply, even if it means avoiding problem areas that may benefit from deep-tissue massage. Once you have a sense of how your body responds to massage, you can slowly experiment with deep-tissue massage. As you begin to recover from fibromyalgia, deep-tissue massage can help your muscles heal from years of inactivity and increased tension. Keep in mind that your dopamine level and corresponding pain sensitivity can vary day to day as your triggers vary. Remember to take it easy during flares. If you're having severe pain, it may be best to take a hot bath or even ice sore muscles and postpone a massage. When you feel better, you can go back to the massage table and get some relief.

When you are lying on a massage table, it's important that you feel comfortable telling the practitioner if the pressure is too intense. You should never feel pain or discomfort on the massage table. If you suffer in silence, you will pay the consequences the next day. Drinking plenty of water before and after your massage will hydrate your body and help flush out any toxins released by the massage. It will also decrease any postmassage soreness you might otherwise experience. Taking a hot bath after your massage may also help the muscles continue to relax. Keep in mind that massage is most beneficial if you are able to do it on a regular basis. Massage is rarely covered by health insurance, so you probably will have to pay for it out of pocket. Regardless, it is still better to pay more money for an experienced practitioner than to spend less for an inexperienced practitioner.

Clinical Findings

A 1999 study in Sweden examined the benefits of massage for fibromyalgia patients. Participants received a series of fifteen massage treatments during a ten-week period. Researchers observed a gradual improvement in the participants' symptoms. At the end of the study, participants experienced a significant reduction in pain. Researchers also observed that massage improved mood, reduced the use of analgesics, and positively affected quality of life. Once the treatment stopped, benefits were relatively short-lived. Three months after the treatment period, about 30 percent of the pain-relieving effect was gone, and after six months, the participants had almost returned to baseline levels of pain.

Osteopathic Manipulation

Although we often think of doctors as MDs (doctors of medicine), some physicians receive their training as DOs (doctors of osteopathy). Doctors of osteopathy attend four years of osteopathic medical school, followed by residency and possibly additional training as specialists. On receiving board certification, an osteopath has the same rights, privileges, and expertise as a medical doctor. The gentle nature of most osteopathic manipulations make it an ideal choice for fibromyalgia patients with underlying physical problems. Unlike many other treatment options described in this section, visits to osteopathic physicians are generally covered by health insurance.

Osteopathic medicine operates off the principle that all of the body's systems work together, and disturbances in one system may affect function elsewhere in the body. Some osteopathic physicians practice osteopathic manipulation, a full-body system of hands-on techniques to alleviate pain, restore function, and promote health and well-being. Osteopathic manipulations are gentle in nature, incorporating rhythmic movements and mild stretches that can help release muscle tension, improve flexibility, stimulate nerves, and improve a joint's range of motion.

Osteopathic physicians generally take a holistic approach to healthcare. If you are unable to find a medical doctor to help with your recovery plan, you should consider finding an osteopathic physician who is willing to help you as you work toward recovery. Unlike medical doctors, many osteopaths are used to seeing patients one or even two times per week to provide physical manipulations. An osteopath can diagnose underlying health problems, write prescriptions, refer you to other specialists, and help work out any underlying physical problems you might have. An osteopath can evaluate all your health needs and provide you with hands-on care. The number of visits needed to experience relief will depend entirely on your body. However, you should notice a difference after two or three physical manipulations. Your osteopath will determine how often you need to be seen.

Clinical Findings

A research team at the University of North Texas Health Science Center studied the benefits of osteopathic manipulation on a small group of fibromyalgia patients. Participants in the study received one osteopathic treatment per week for six months. Participants who received osteopathic manipulation had significantly higher pain thresholds at the end of the study. They were also reported to be significantly more satisfied, more comfortable, more relaxed, and less strained when compared with patients not receiving the same treatment. They also reported fewer symptoms related to failure, frustration, inhibition, struggling, helplessness, guilt, incapacity, wakefulness, and tiredness associated with pain. Overall, researchers found that the use of osteopathic manipulation raised pain thresholds, improved comfort levels, and increased the perceived functional abilities of treated patients.

Chiropractic Treatments

Millions of Americans visit chiropractors every year for the treatment of back pain, neck pain, headaches, sports injuries, repetitive strains, and other problems generally associated with poor alignment of the musculoskeletal system. A chiropractor is a licensed healthcare professional who has received extensive chiropractic training. Chiropractic training involves a four-year academic program involving classroom and clinical instruction. Chiropractors use hands-on manipulation to treat problems with the muscles, joints, bones, and connective tissues. Chiropractors use a wide variety of manipulative techniques that range from subtle to forceful. Chiropractors may also use other techniques, such as the application of heat and ice, ultrasound, electrical stimulation, rehabilitative exercise, and magnetic therapy.

Chiropractic manipulation is the most commonly used form of alternative medicine in the United States. This structural approach to healing may help relieve acute or chronic pain in the back or other areas. It may also help relieve pain caused by trigger points or cervical spine stenosis. As is the case with all other treatments, you should choose a provider who is familiar with fibromyalgia. A chiropractic session should not cause pain or discomfort. Chiropractic work is often covered by health insurance and may be covered by Medicare and Medicaid. Many plans limit the number of visits covered and/or require that you see a chiropractor in their network.

Chiropractors practice a wide range of techniques, and anyone you see will have his or her own style. Some chiropractors use extremely gentle techniques, while others use more forceful manipulations. If you don't like the first chiropractor you visit, don't necessarily rule out this therapy. Check around and find someone who has a technique that works well with your personality and physical needs. Once a chiropractor has evaluated your condition, he or she will determine how often you should be seen. You may start out seeing a chiropractor twice a week and then go down to once a week if you start feeling better. Like most other therapies, you should notice a difference within two or three visits if chiropractic care is going to offer any true relief for your body.

If you have osteoporosis, rheumatoid arthritis, sciatica, or other painful underlying conditions, consult with your doctor before seeking chiropractic care. In some cases, spinal manipulations could aggravate your existing condition.

Clinical Findings

Two small studies have found that chiropractic treatment may help reduce pain and improve range of motion for fibromyalgia patients. One of the studies found that treatments were more likely to be effective for younger patients with fewer symptoms. The study found that in general, older patients with higher levels of chronic pain did not respond to chiropractic treatment. One of the studies also found a corresponding improvement in quality of sleep and fatigue level after fifteen treatments.

Physical Therapy

Physical therapy combines a wide range of therapies and techniques to help rebuild muscle strength, release tight muscles and trigger points, restore range of motion in joints and muscles, and heal damage caused by an injury. Physical therapy presents a multilayered approach that can be extremely beneficial for fibromyalgia patients. Physical therapists use many different therapeutic approaches, including massage, exercise, ultrasound, electrical stimulation, light therapy, traction, and heat and cold treatments. Physical therapy may benefit your body by helping to resolve underlying physical problems or by helping you slowly regain strength and function that has been lost over time.

As you know, with fibromyalgia, even a modest injury can be completely disabling due to your amplified pain signals. If you have an underlying injury or another physical problem such as tendonitis, a good physical therapist can help resolve this problem and eliminate one of your sources of pain. Remember—all the pain you feel is real, and if some of it stems from an underlying injury or aggravation, it can be resolved with appropriate treatment. A skilled physical therapist who has experience with fibromyalgia patients can help determine whether an underlying problem may be causing some of your pain.

If you have suffered from fibromyalgia for a long time, some of your muscles may have atrophied due to lack of use. A physical therapist can guide you through an exercise program designed to gently stretch and strengthen unused muscles, helping you regain any of the physical functions you may have lost. Over time, you may have also unconsciously developed poor posture in an attempt to protect different parts of your body from too much movement. Poor body posture or body mechanics can create a whole new set of problems for your body to contend with. A physical therapist can also help you with your posture, teaching you how to carry yourself in a way that minimizes stress on your joints and muscles.

Physical therapy has a proven track record of helping people recover from both minor and traumatic physical problems. If you are considering physical therapy, take the time to find a physical therapist who understands how to work with fibromyalgia patients. If you are looking for a physical therapist to treat an underlying physical injury, find someone who specializes in treating that type of injury. There are many different approaches to physical therapy, and it may take you more than one try to find the right physical therapist for your body.

You will generally need a referral from your primary care physician to see a physical therapist. Your primary care physician will first diagnose the underlying physical problem and then prescribe a course of physical therapy. A course of physical therapy generally involves two to three visits a week over a four- to six-week period. If the therapy is helping, your physician can extend your prescription at the end of the initial time frame. Most health insurance plans cover physical therapy, but be sure to read the specifics of your plan. Without health insurance, physical therapy is an expensive treatment option.

Acupuncture

Acupuncture has been a mainstay of Chinese medicine for over two thousand years, making it one of the oldest and most commonly used medical treatments in the world. For several decades, increasing numbers of Americans have turned to acupuncture for help with relieving chronic pain, migraines, fatigue, allergies, nausea, and many other problems not easily resolved by Western medicine. I was surprised, at first, to learn that many of my patients had tried acupuncture in an effort to find symptom relief. Although they reported mixed results, I have encountered more than a few patients who reported positive experiences with acupuncture.

Chinese medicine is based on the belief that health problems result from an imbalance in the body's energy flow along pathways known as meridians. The goal of acupuncture is to rebalance the flow of energy, or qi, in the body by stimulating specific acupuncture points on the skin. An acupuncturist carefully inserts long, thin needles just below the skin in order to stimulate these points. Not all acupuncturists use needles—electroacupuncture, pressure, and laser-generated light treatments are also used to stimulate these points. Although it sounds painful, most people don't even feel the tiny needles as they enter the top layer of skin.

Scientists are not entirely sure how acupuncture works, but the evidence seems to be mounting that in some cases, acupuncture helps ease pain and speed healing. Western scientists studying acupuncture believe that the treatment may help regulate the central nervous system (CNS), stimulating the activity of painkilling endorphins and immune system cells at specific sites. Some studies have shown that acupuncture effects the release of neurotransmitters and neurohormones by the CNS and therefore may influence pain and other sensations. If this is true, acupuncture may offer some benefits for fibromyalgia patients. Unlike the other therapies described in this chapter, you do not necessarily need to visit an acupuncturist for a specific physical problem. You can visit an acupuncturist for any of your general symptoms or in an attempt to slow down the fight-or-flight response in your body.

As strange as it may seem, many people find acupuncture extremely relaxing. Some even fall asleep during their treatments, which can last for fifteen to forty-five minutes. If you decide to try acupuncture, be sure to visit a licensed practitioner. In addition to traditional acupuncturists, more and more medical doctors, osteopaths, and other Western practitioners are cross-training in acupuncture and offering it to their patients. In some cases, acupuncture is covered by health insurance plans. Acupuncture generally involves several sessions, and results, if any, may not be apparent after just one or two sessions. However, you should notice some difference after four or five sessions if acupuncture is going to provide relief.

If you believe that acupuncture will help you, then by all means, give it a try. Sometimes, the power of believing that you are taking care of your body can have a remarkable healing effect all by itself. On top of that, acupuncture might provide some relief as well.

Clinical Findings

Studies on the efficacy of acupuncture for easing fibromyalgia symptoms have produced mixed results. Several studies indicate that acupuncture may be beneficial for short-term pain relief. A study at the Mayo Clinic investigated whether acupuncture would help the symptoms of moderate to severe fibromyalgia for patients who hadn't found relief from other treatments. After six sessions of acupuncture over a two- to three-week period, participants in the study experienced short-term improvements in pain, fatigue, and anxiety. Several other studies have reported benefits for fibromyalgia patients, although one study found no difference between real acupuncture and acupuncture that didn't stimulate real acupuncture points. Most studies have been of relatively short duration and did not follow patients for a significant period of time to determine whether any long-term benefits existed.

Trigger-Point Therapy

Trigger points can be an underlying cause of debilitating pain in fibromyalgia patients. Trigger points and tender points are not the same thing. Tender points are specific areas in the body that are extremely sensitive to pressure. To some extent, everyone has tender points if these areas are pushed on hard enough. With fibromyalgia, you become extremely aware of your tender points. Trigger points are different. A trigger point can result from an injury or the repetitive use of a muscle group. Located in taut bands of muscle, these pea-size lumps not only cause excruciating pain at the site of the trigger point but refer pain to other areas as well.

Trigger points are either latent or active. An active trigger point causes pain, while a latent trigger point may restrict movement or cause weakness. Either way, trigger points can make fibromyalgia even more miserable. You don't have to wonder whether you have trigger points. They are easily identified through palpations by a physician or physical therapist with experience in this area. Trigger points can be released through massage, acupressure, physical therapy techniques, and injections. The pain of trigger points can sometimes be alleviated through heat and ice treatments.

Trigger-point injections are one of the most effective ways to release these painfully constricted areas. Unfortunately, the actual treatment can also be pretty unpleasant for someone already suffering from amplified pain sensations. Trigger-point injections should only be performed by a physician. After locating the trigger point, a physician inserts a needle directly into this painful spot. The needle itself interrupts the trigger point and stimulates its release. Sometimes physicians also inject a small amount of numbing lidocaine, but it is the action of the needle stimulating the trigger point that results in relief. If you have moderate to severe fibromyalgia, you may want to try less invasive options for treating your trigger points. The procedure itself can produce short-term stiffness and pain in the treated area. However, if you can tolerate this procedure, it can produce immediate and lasting results. Trigger-point injections are most effective when followed by massage.

Finding a Practitioner

Complementary therapies can be extremely helpful in your battle against fibromyalgia. Anything that makes you feel better in the short term will put you one step closer to long-term recovery. However, use caution as you explore complementary therapies. Don't expect any particular therapy to provide a "cure." In fact, be suspicious of anyone who promises to solve the fibromyalgia problem for you. Only you can do that. If you have misgivings at any point, ask yourself, "Is this worth it? Is it worth my time and money? Is it too painful? Is it too risky? Can I really trust this person?" Never be afraid to change your mind, no matter how far along in the treatment you are.

In order to get the most for your time and money, you'll want to spend some time researching the best practitioner for you. If you have a good relationship with your primary care physician, discuss any options you are considering with him or her first. He or she may have a list of practitioners other patients have used, with good results. In some cases, a prescription from your primary care physician for massage, physical therapy, or other therapies may be necessary in order for your health insurance to cover the additional costs.

Talk to friends or relatives who have personal experience with some of these options. Get their referrals, recommendations, and especially their advice on who *not* to see. If you know other people with fibromyalgia, they may be excellent sources of information. It is important to choose a practitioner who is familiar with fibromyalgia. You need someone to understand that your body is different from those of most of their clients and that you may need a lighter or more gentle approach in the beginning.

Take into consideration the costs of different treatments. If your health insurance doesn't cover a specific type of therapy or the practitioner you want to see, talk to the provider about the cost of the treatment before your first visit. He or she may offer a sliding scale of payments depending on your income or may be willing to work with you if you need to make install-ment payments.

Prior to making an appointment, be sure you feel comfortable with the practitioner you are seeing and the type of treatment he or she offers. Within any particular therapy type, there is a wide range of philosophies, and treatments may vary widely from one practitioner to the next. When you contact a practitioner's office, ask what training or other qualifications the practi-tioner has. Find out how long he or she has been practicing and whether the practitioner has any specialized training related to the problem you are experiencing. Ask, in particular, whether the practitioner commonly treats people with fibromyalgia. If possible, ask to speak with the provider by phone before making an appointment. In most cases, people are more than willing to speak with you for a few moments.

Ask the practitioner whether he or she is familiar with fibromyalgia and how he or she might adjust the treatment for someone with fibromyalgia. Ask whether the practitioner believes the treatment can help provide relief for your particular problem. Also, ask the practitioner how many patients he or she typically sees in a day and how much time he or she typically spends with each patient. You should also ask what to expect during your first session and how many treatments might be needed to relieve your condition.

If you feel comfortable with the answers to these questions and the practitioner has good references and the appropriate credentials, you may have found the right person for your body. If the practitioner does not call you back or does not have time to answer questions prior to an appointment, he or she might not be the right person for you. If you do make an appointment, be sure to spend some time at the first appointment discussing your body and any concerns you might have about the treatment. If you feel at any time that a treatment may be doing more harm than good, listen to your intuition. Before you begin your first session, be sure you feel comfortable telling a practitioner to stop or slow down. At the end of the session, ask what you might expect to feel the next day, especially in light of your fibromyalgia.

In a Nutshell . . .

- Complementary therapies can help you resolve any underlying physical problems that contribute to your pain.
- Complementary therapies won't necessarily heal you, but they may speed up the healing process.
- Many therapies have proven track records with helping fibromyalgia sufferers reduce their pain and other symptoms.
- Complementary therapies should never cause you pain.
- Use care when choosing a provider. Find someone who has worked with fibromyalgia patients before, and avoid anyone who claims to be able to cure fibromyalgia.

CHAPTER 12

Moving Beyond Fibromyalgia

By now, you should have a much better idea of what fibromyalgia is, how it can affect you, and what you can do about it. Although you may feel inspired, inspiration alone won't get you to the finish line. Recovering from fibromyalgia takes a systematic, step-by-step approach. As we discussed, creating a case history, identifying your physical and psychological triggers, and working with your doctor to resolve underlying medical conditions will allow you to develop a long-term recovery plan.

Don't plan your recovery in your head only. Put your plan on paper in your Progress Journal, and be very specific about the steps you need to take to reverse the fibromyalgia cycle. If you feel stuck and even the recovery plan seems overwhelming, just make a list of everything that may be currently triggering your fight-or-flight response and depleting dopamine. Then, make a list of everything you can think of that might improve your situation. Don't be daunted by the size or scope of your list. There's no need to be overly ambitious and take on all your fibromyalgia triggers at once. Anything you do to slow down your fight-or-flight response and boost your dopamine levels, no matter how small, is a step in the right direction. If you can only pick one thing to work on at a time, you'll still make progress. Of course, the more you can successfully take on, the faster your recovery. Now, let's take a look at a real-life success story.

A Success Story

Tom has a soft voice and Santa Claus eyes that twinkle when he talks. Tom laughs a lot, but that's a recent development. Most people grow older and discover pain. In Tom's case, he has lived with pain his entire life. It was only on approaching his seventieth birthday that Tom discovered what it was like to live without pain.

Tom was born bow-legged due to a curvature of the bones in his legs. Doctors told his mother that he would probably never walk. It was 1935, the middle of the Depression, and his family didn't have any money for leg braces. During the first year of his life, his mother had to manually straighten his legs each day, which was an extremely painful process for Tom. He grew up on a little farm in rural Missouri on the edge of Grandview. His parents were both alcoholics, and he didn't always know where they were. Living with alcoholic parents forced Tom to grow up very quickly. In the absence of his parents, Tom found himself taking care of his brothers and sisters. Before long, he developed a very sensitive fight-or-flight response.

Tom grew up in a lot of pain. The pain started in his legs but then moved throughout his body. Some of it was a physical, structural pain related to the problems with his legs. Some of the pain moved around and was hard to understand. For a long time, he thought everybody's bodies were like this.

At around fourteen or fifteen years old, he discovered through casual conversation that not everyone lived in pain. It came as quite a shock to learn how different he was.

Tom saw many doctors over the years, and they always gave him a blank stare. The doctors told him that there was no physical reason for his pain, and Tom began to think he was crazy. Finally, Tom gave up on talking to doctors and accepted pain as his ordeal in life. Over the years, he learned to live with the pain, but sometimes he would break down and cry. Sports were out of the question, running became too painful, and his life became more sedentary. He tried skiing for a while, but the problem was that falling hurt *a lot*. Other people would fall and get right back up, but when he fell, it would hurt for days. Finally, he couldn't ignore the pain anymore.

Things changed when Tom was in his sixties, when he found a primary care doctor who was interested in hearing what he had to say and trying to figure out what was wrong. He was the first doctor to really care, to want to help Tom get rid of his pain. He suspected fibromyalgia and referred Tom to me. Tom clearly had fibromyalgia. He had an underlying medical cause—the structural problem in his legs—and he had his feisty Irish temper, which I explained was another name for an overactive fight-or-flight response.

At that first visit, I talked to Tom about controlling his fight-or-flight response. He immediately understood what I was talking about. I also started him on Mirapex in hope of controlling his symptoms as soon as possible. I figured that after sixty-six years of pain, I would have to pull out all the stops to help Tom. He is one of the lucky ones, if it's possible to say that about somebody who has suffered from pain his entire life. But, with regard to Mirapex, Tom had no trouble taking the medication.

When I saw Tom at his follow-up visit, I was amazed. His pain was reduced by approximately 80 to 90 percent. Ninety percent of the battle, he said, was simply knowing what was wrong. Once he understood that there was a rational reason for his pain and possibly a cure, Tom got serious about working on all his fibromyalgia triggers. He learned how to control his fight-or-flight response, and he scheduled two painful knee surgeries to correct the structural problems in his legs. For the first time in his life, he could stand on straight legs. Although his pain was almost gone, his primary care physician decided to try Cymbalta, an antidepressant that affects serotonin and norepinephrine. With the addition of Cymbalta, Tom's pain disappeared entirely.

Today, Tom is pain-free. He attributes his success to four things:

1. My approach and explanation of fibromyalgia
2. Taking Mirapex
3. Learning more about the fight-or-flight response through my seminars, counseling, and Al-Anon (a support group for the friends and family members of alcoholics)
4. Taking Cymbalta for the remaining pain in his body

Tom emphasizes that it is more than just pain that has changed in his life. Mentally, he is in a different place. He keeps his Irish temper in check, and both he and his family are happier for it. He drove to Colorado recently, and the car died in Wyoming. He was stranded there for two days but stayed calm the entire time. "That is simply not me," says Tom. Tom has renewed physical and mental health. He says the two are so intertwined, it is hard to have one without the other. Tom says, "I'm the person I really want to be. I don't stress. I don't involve myself in other people's affairs. It is a new type of freedom."

The most important part of Tom's success is that he worked on everything that could be contributing to fibromyalgia. He went to counseling to control his fight-or-flight response, and he attended all my seminars on the topic. He sought out surgery to correct an underlying medical problem. He also took Mirapex and Cymbalta to aid the process of recovery. Even without these medications, I think Tom would still have recovered from fibromyalgia because of his dedication to the recovery process.

Everyday Obstacles

Everyone wants to recover from fibromyalgia, and everyone starts out with good intentions. The difference between recovery and failure lies in your ability to overcome the obstacles that get in the way of your best intentions. Listed below are some of the most common obstacles people face and how to overcome them:

I don't have the time. You can't expect your recovery to just happen. You will have to make time for it, which may mean making changes to your daily or weekly routine. Finding enough time to heal is one of the biggest stumbling blocks for a lot of my patients. I'll ask you the same question I ask everyone else: What would you sacrifice now in order to feel great and have energy for the rest of your life? Would you take a break from your job? Would you borrow money? Would you ask a friend to take care of your kids once a week? Would you move into a smaller house? Many people have to make hard choices now in order to secure a happy and healthy future.

When people have fibromyalgia, they try desperately to maintain a semblance of their former lives. Everyone has a fear that if they start letting go of different things, their lives will never be the same. You have to stop believing that you're going to be sick forever. If you can take the time out for yourself now, no matter how hard it seems, you'll have infinitely more time to accomplish anything you need to for the rest of your life. Don't imagine for a moment that you are being selfish. If you can give yourself some extra time now and allow your body to heal, you're giving everyone else the greatest gift you can: your health.

I don't have enough energy for this. If you feel like you're out of energy, start small. Find someone who will encourage you and help you get started. Work on improving things that will give you more energy. Do you need to improve your sleep? Could your diet be healthier? Take small but productive steps that are guaranteed to increase your energy level. Although the initial outpouring of physical and mental energy may seem like a lot, the payoff will be worth it.

I don't have enough money. As long as you don't have untreated medical causes that need attention, such as sleep apnea, the most effective way to resolve fibromyalgia doesn't have to cost a lot. There are many different ways to attack fibromyalgia. Money can make it easier if it allows you to take time off from work or to treat underlying causes with physical therapy. However, a lack of money should never stand in your way. Some of my wealthiest patients have spent tens of thousands of dollars trying to resolve fibromyalgia only to discover that the real cure comes from within.

Nobody believes me. Many patients tell me that most of the people in their lives simply scoff at the idea of fibromyalgia. Some people have even come to believe that fibromyalgia is nothing more than the diagnosis physicians trot out when they have no idea what's going on with a patient. In the past, there may have been some truth to that.

The better you understand your own case of fibromyalgia, the more likely it is that you will be able to explain it clearly to the people around you. Unfortunately, even as you come to grips with fibromyalgia, its underpinnings, and its implications, it still may be difficult to convince some of the people around you of what's happening to you. Sadly, this could include your primary healthcare provider, who actually may know very little about fibromyalgia or, more likely, may be relying on outdated thinking. Don't let other people's opinions get in the way of your recovery. Fibromyalgia is real, and it's your battle to win or lose—not theirs.

I can't avoid stress. In today's chaotic world, no one can avoid stressful situations, but you can always do a better job of avoiding the harmful effects of stress. If you can easily identify your fight-or-flight response but can't seem to control it, don't give up. A good counselor can help you work on controlling the fight-or-flight response. You can also check out my Web site for upcoming seminars, workshops, and even teleconferences on learning more about fibromyalgia and the fight-or-flight response: www.drdryland.com.

I can't find a doctor who will help me. A lot of people have trouble finding a good doctor who won't write them off once they mention fibromyalgia. Throughout the medical community, there still remains a broad divergence of beliefs regarding what fibromyalgia is actually all about. Some physicians discount its existence altogether. Others care for their fibromyalgia patients appropriately but are still waiting for better treatment options to become available. Others simply ascribe their patients' problems to nothing more than depression.

Much of the work you need to accomplish can be done on your own, but it's extremely helpful to have a supportive physician. One of my hopes in writing this book is to change minds and attitudes about fibromyalgia. I believe that once physicians understand what fibromyalgia is and how to effectively help people, they will be more willing to work with people like you. If you don't have any underlying medical causes, you should be fine on your own. If you do have other medical conditions, find a doctor to treat those conditions. You can do the rest yourself!

I'm in a really stressful relationship. Stressful relationships are one of the most common obstacles my patients face. A difficult relationship can drive your adrenaline levels through the roof. Fibromyalgia generally makes things worse, especially if your partner doesn't seem supportive. As you go through the life-changing process of recovering from fibromyalgia, you can use this relationship as an opportunity to work on controlling your fight-or-flight response. Remember, don't blame others for your own insecurities. If you choose to leave the relationship, you may be giving up one of the best opportunities to erase a lot of misguided security needs. In the end, the hard work you do could successfully change the dynamics of the relationship for the better. If not, you'll know when it's time to leave. I never advise people to stay in relationships if they are suffering physical abuse. This is not the time to apply the triad—it's time to leave and get help.

Nothing seems to help. What if you follow the recommendations in this book and some of your symptoms improve, but you still have fibromyalgia? You probably need to review your list of triggers. Is it possible you've overlooked one? Or did you just fail to see something you didn't want to see? I've had patients, for example, who really needed back surgery, but—for one reason or another—kept putting it off. Well, it turns out that part of the price they ended up paying for that was an intense case of fibromyalgia. In other instances, I've found that a key contributing trigger had to do with the fact that a patient was putting off some dreaded decision—for example, whether to put an elderly parent into a nursing home. The result there, of course, is that all the mounting stress ends up leaving the person stuck in semipermanent fight-or-flight mode. This is exactly why I urge everyone who thinks they might be wrestling with psychological causes (including stress) to take the time to learn how to properly tone down their fight-or-flight response.

So what are your obstacles to success? Don't let them hide in the recesses of your mind, where they will get in the way of your recovery. Write them down in your Progress Journal, where you can see them in broad daylight. By acknowledging them, you can be proactive about overcoming them. Talk to other people about your obstacles, and brainstorm the different ways you can surmount them.

Develop a Support System

Recovering from fibromyalgia is a challenging journey and one that is extremely difficult, if not impossible, to do on your own. As you are drafting your recovery plan, think about the people you want to include on your recovery team. You'll continue to have bad days as well as good days, and you will need a group of people who understand your plan and are there to help you see it through. Share your recovery plan with these people. Let them know you're serious about getting better and that you need help. If possible, find one person who is willing to check in with you on a weekly basis. On good weeks, you'll want someone who can appreciate your successes, and on challenging weeks, you'll want someone who can listen to your frustration.

It can be hard to ask for help, but most people feel better about themselves when they are able to help someone else in a positive and constructive way. So don't be shy. Ask for help. Do you need someone to walk with? a babysitter? someone to help you shop for and cook nutritious food? People will be excited to help you when they know you have a concrete recovery plan. Once they understand that they are helping you recover, they'll be even more excited to get on board.

You can also look for support outside your family and friends. As I have already noted, if at all possible, it will be extremely helpful to have a good physician on your side. Find someone who is open-minded and willing to work with you on resolving underlying medical causes, prescribing medication when needed, and monitoring your overall health as you move beyond fibromyalgia. As we discussed in chapter 7, another important person in your recovery may be a therapist or counselor. A good therapist or counselor can help you overcome mental obstacles getting in the way of your recovery. I also recommend finding a fibromyalgia support group as you work toward recovery. People with fibromyalgia will appreciate your struggles and be impressed by your successes like no one else. It's also helpful to connect with other people who are working toward recovery. As I mentioned earlier, I created an online support group called The Forum to provide support for people like you. Members share stories of recovery, both good and bad, and offer personal advice from their own experiences. It's a great place to get to know people who have a common goal—moving beyond fibromyalgia. You can sign up for The Forum on my Web site: www.drdryland.com. You can also register for my e-newsletter, *Freedom from Fibromyalgia,* and stay in touch with the latest information on fibromyalgia, controlling the fight-or-flight response, seminars, workshops, support groups, and other happenings in your area.

Explaining Fibromyalgia

In order to generate support from friends, family members, coworkers, and even physicians, you'll need to explain how fibromyalgia works. Even armed with your new knowledge, it can still be a challenge to explain fibromyalgia to the rest of the world. Although many people have heard the word "fibromyalgia" and often nod their heads to indicate understanding when they hear it again, they would be hard-pressed to describe the condition. Also, because there is no visible body damage, others may question whether you're truly suffering. They may think you're faking or that you're simply imagining aches and pains. Often, I've witnessed the anguish caused by doubts raised by loved ones and friends. It is important to remember that people can be made uncomfortable by things they do not understand.

Since fibromyalgia has been misdiagnosed and misunderstood for so many years, your challenge is to clearly explain what it really means to have the condition. In doing so, you will provide your friends, loved ones, and healthcare providers with the tools they need to help you work toward a cure. Sharing information about your condition can be empowering for everyone involved.

You can explain fibromyalgia through science-based explanations, physical demonstrations, and by sharing your thoughts and feelings. Your personality or the personalities of those around you will help you determine which approach to choose.

Explaining Fibromyalgia Through Science

The primary reason fibromyalgia is so misunderstood is because people do not understand the science behind it. I've found that once I provide people with a physiological explanation of how fibromyalgia works, they suddenly become much more interested and empathetic. Here are some suggestions you can use to explain fibromyalgia:

- Fibromyalgia is not a disease but a very painful and potentially chronic condition that people can develop in association with great amounts of psychological or physical stress.
- The brain cannot tell the difference between physical and emotional pain. In either situation, the brain activates the fight-or-flight response and floods the body with adrenaline and other stress hormones. Increased adrenaline levels cause changes in your body, allowing you to run faster, fight harder, and focus more clearly on the situation at hand.
- Dopamine, another stress hormone, plays an important role in the fight-or-flight response. Dopamine effectively blocks the painful sensations that might otherwise keep you from running to safety on an injured leg. Dopamine also plays an important role in filtering everyday sensations. But when you have fibromyalgia, you have low levels of dopamine, and thus you continually experience more pain.
- Due to its dependency on stress hormones, the fight-or-flight response was meant to be used in true emergencies. When you have fibromyalgia, the fight-or-flight response is continually overactivated.
- Once your dopamine is depleted, increased pain levels continue to trigger the fight-or-flight response, creating a vicious cycle.

- Fibromyalgia is curable and does not directly damage the body. However, the pain and symptoms caused by fibromyalgia can be almost unbearable at times.
- Recovery depends on a person's ability to identify and resolve his or her fibromyalgia triggers.

Depending on who you are talking to, you may want to add your own examples and explain the triggers that are unique to your case of fibromyalgia.

Explaining Fibromyalgia Through Physical Demonstrations

One good way to explain fibromyalgia is to show your friends and family how to identify their own tender points (see chapter 5, figure 9). Tender points are naturally sensitive areas that can become extremely painful once the fibromyalgia cycle is triggered. Ask your friends and loved ones to apply pressure to their own tender points. Is the pressure uncomfortable? Can they tell that we all have a lot of sensitive areas in our bodies? If so, you can explain that you live with these sensations, greatly amplified, all over your body . . . every second of every day.

You'll also want people to understand that you are sensitive to more than just pain. Ask your friends to remember the last time they were in a dimly lit or otherwise darkened room for a while, when suddenly the whole room was lit by the bright flash of a camera. Can they remember how everyone moaned and shielded their eyes from the offending flash? The sensitivity that their unprepared eyes experienced during that brief moment is similar to the sensitivity continually experienced by fibromyalgia patients. If they want to know what it's like to experience other amplified sensations, ask them to wear an item of clothing that continually irritates their skin.

It could be an irritating seam, a misplaced tag, or the mere texture of the clothing. Each of these irritations is probably enough to keep them from wearing that piece of clothing very often. Explain that all of your sensations are heightened in a similar way all the time.

Explaining Fibromyalgia by Sharing Thoughts and Feelings

In relationships where you have already developed an emotional connection, one of the easiest ways to explain fibromyalgia is to share your thoughts, feelings, and experiences. Ask your loved ones to think back to the last time they had the flu. Did they feel like having sex? How much interest did they have in going out to the movies? Was it easy to get up in the morning to see the kids off to school? Chances are, they stayed in bed as much as they could, making only the occasional outing to the bathroom or kitchen. It might have been days before they even thought of leaving the house. Ask them if they can imagine functioning on a day-to-day basis with those symptoms. Explain to them that you don't have the luxury of taking those days off, because sometimes every day feels like one of those days.

Fibromyalgia in the Workplace

In addition to your friends and loved ones, you may also want to explain your fibromyalgia to your employer. Fibromyalgia can dramatically affect your ability to be productive at work. If your employer or direct supervisor understands your condition, he or she may be able to help you create less stressful working conditions with the mutual goal of once again having a highly productive employee. Prior to talking with your employer, make a list of the ways you are still productive in your job. Make a secondary list of reasonable accommodations that would allow you to be more productive in your job. These could include:

- allowing a self-paced workload and flexible hours
- allowing you to work from home
- providing a part-time work schedule
- creating an ergonomically correct work space
- allowing time for medical appointments

In addition to improving your performance, your employer may also be eligible for tax deductions or business credits, depending on the type of accommodation it makes. If your employer is covered by the employment provisions of the Americans with Disabilities Act (ADA), it is prohibited from discriminating against qualified individuals with disabilities. The following resources can provide you with more information on these topics:

ADA Information Center: 800-949-4232
Job Accommodation Network: 800-526-7234

When talking with your employer, the most important goal to work toward is the creation of a work environment that will benefit both of you.

If you are attempting to obtain disability compensation, you may be in for some rough sledding. In 1999, the U.S. Social Security Administration included fibromyalgia in its list of disabling conditions. However, this does not mean that everyone with fibromyalgia will be determined to be disabled. That's because a healthcare provider relies chiefly on the patient's symptoms to make a diagnosis of fibromyalgia.

However, insurance companies and disability review boards would rather see objective data—namely, findings from physical exams, lab reports, radiological scans, surgical reports, or any other measurable findings.

Let's imagine that you developed fibromyalgia in part because of the stress you endure as an air-traffic controller. First of all, where's the hard data to support your claim of fibromyalgia? Second, how can you prove that stress from your work environment helped to bring it on? And finally, how can you convince a skeptical supervisor that your current condition interferes with your ability to perform your job? Chances are that people will question your story. In part, that's because people are uncomfortable and rather unforgiving when it comes to understanding any condition that may have a mental or psychological dimension. In our society, the mere mention of anxiety or depression can often be viewed as a sign of weakness.

This may be changing, as more and more research confirms my findings regarding fibromyalgia. For example, there now is indisputable scientific evidence that chronic stress or interrupted sleep leads to amplified pain sensations. Over time, it's likely that much of the rest of my diagnostic criteria will also come to be more commonly accepted and recognized. And that should make the evaluation of fibromyalgia much more straightforward for everyone—including disability review boards.

Don't Just Get Better, Get Healthy

If you follow even some of the recommendations in this book with any dedication, your symptoms will improve. Some people are tempted to be satisfied with simply feeling better.

Don't lose sight of the long-term goal—moving beyond fibromyalgia forever. Many of the recommendations in this book will help reduce your symptoms, but there's only one way to really get past fibromyalgia. You have to go directly after the matter that's at the root of all your other problems—namely, your overactive fight-or-flight response.

Keep in mind that even the most diligent work on your triggers is not going to yield a quick fix. That's because this work is a slow and steady process, not an event. It is important to remember that the longer you've suffered with the effects of increased adrenaline, the longer it's going to take your brain to unlearn its reflexive fight-or-flight way of responding to the outside world. This is why you may find that improvements come slowly, even if you happen to be making excellent progress in terms of working on your triggers. That's when it will be important to remind yourself that even though the improvements may be small, they're long-term improvements. You're in the process of rebalancing your autonomic nervous system, thus allowing it to operate correctly again for perhaps the first time in many years.

Fibromyalgia begins and ends with the fight-or-flight response. At any given moment, your brain can decide that a particular situation merits extra adrenaline. You will then feel an overwhelming urge to think or do something about a perceived problem. It will be impossible to free your brain's grip on your life without dealing with the way you use the fight-or-flight response. This is why I tell my patients that fibromyalgia is an opportunity—actually the best opportunity of their lives. People who don't suffer from fibromyalgia still often suffer the consequences of an overactive fight-or-flight response. They will rarely make the hard changes that would bring them true happiness. Pain, however, is a powerful motivator. Fibromyalgia essentially forces you to go down this path of finally reining in your fight-or-flight response and gaining true control over your brain. Not only will the pain finally leave you, true happiness will be your eventual reward. Do not settle for anything less.

The amazing part about this program is that you will achieve so much more than recovery from fibromyalgia! Your recovery will force you to improve many aspects of your life. Along the way, you may have to figure out how to overcome some of the biggest challenges you've ever faced. When you're finished, you will not only get your life back, but thanks to all your hard work, it will be better than ever before.

A Note from the Author

As a doctor, I can only see a limited number of patients. When my patients began recovering from fibromyalgia, I suddenly had a lot of doctors, nurses, physical therapists, and other fibromyalgia sufferers wanting to know how they did it. I realized there was a tremendous need to share the good news about fibromyalgia. Soon, I started leading seminars and teaching workshops on fibromyalgia and the fight-or-flight response. This book is one part of my effort to reach out to people who mistakenly believe they suffer from an incurable condition. You can learn more about my work on fibromyalgia and the fight-or-flight response at www.drdryland.com. You can also meet other people who are fighting a similar battle when you join The Forum, an online discussion group for people like you. The Forum allows people to share advice, swap success stories, and ask questions. Sign up for our e-newsletter, *Freedom from Fibromyalgia,* and stay up-to-date on my travel schedule, future seminars, workshop opportunities, and teleconferences.

Recommended Resources

Chapter 6: Sleeping Well

Books

This is a must-read for anyone who suffers from insomnia: *Say Good Night to Insomnia* by Gregg Jacobs.

Organizations/Web Sites

The National Sleep Foundation offers a free, interactive sleep diary and many other useful resources: www.national sleepfoundation.org.

For a wealth of information, including articles on the latest sleep research, links to helpful Web sites, and updates on prescription medications, check out MedlinePlus, a Web site sponsored by the National Library of Medicine and the National Institutes of Health: www.nlm.nih.gov/medlineplus/ sleepdisorders.html, or go to www.medlineplus.gov and enter "sleep" in the search box.

For more information on sleep disorders, including detailed information on prescription sleeping medications, visit www.medicinenet.com/sleep/focus.htm.

Northside Hospital Sleep Medicine Institute offers an online test designed to help people recognize and detect symptoms of sleep disorders: www.nshsleep.com.

The American Sleep Apnea Association Web site has information on sleep apnea, including a link to support groups throughout the country: www.sleepapnea.org.

The Restless Legs Syndrome Foundation provides information on RLS as well as links to support groups: www.rls.org.

Chapter 7: Reducing Stress—Easier Said Than Done

Videos

If you want to learn more about your fight-or-flight response and how to control it, I recommend watching my DVD seminar: *Taking Control of Your Fight or Flight Response,* which is available at my Web site: www.drdryland.com. Also available is *Further Lessons on the Fight or Flight Response,* a follow-up audio CD set that takes the lessons in the DVD seminar one step further.

Books

A great resource for anyone looking to reduce the stress of interpersonal relationships is *Nonviolent Communication: A Language of Life* by Marshall Rosenberg.

For more information on how to meditate, check out the following books:

8 Minute Meditation: Quiet Your Mind. Change Your Life by Victor Davich

Meditation for Beginners: Six Guided Meditations for Insight, Inner Clarity, and Cultivating a Compassionate Heart by Jack Kornfield

Breath by Breath by Larry Rosenberg

CDs

For guidance in practicing meditation, try one of these audio CDs:

Guided Meditations for Stress Reduction by Bodhipaksa
Guided Mediations: For Calmness, Awareness, and Love by Bodhipaksa

Web Sites

You can find more information on the fight-or-flight response on my Web site: www.drdryland.com.

A recommended Web site for improving communication skills is www.nonviolentcommunication.com.

If you think you are suffering from depression, the National Institute of Mental Health provides a lot of good information and helpful links at www.nimh.nih.gov/HealthInformation/depressionmenu.cfm.

The National Mental Health Association offers a confidential depression screening test and information on clinical depression at www.depression-screening.org.

Information on bipolar disorder is available at www.nimh.nih.gov/healthinformation/bipolarmenu.cfm.

Information on anxiety disorder is available at www.nimh.nih.gov/HealthInformation/anxietymenu.cfm.

Information on Posttraumatic stress disorder is available at www.nlm.nih.gov/medlineplus/posttraumaticstressdisorder.html.

Chapter 8: Eating Well and Feeling Better

Working with a Clinical Nutritionist

If you're interested in learning more about tailoring your diet to meet the needs of your body, I recommend consulting a clinical nutritionist (CN). A CN works primarily with individuals to treat or prevent disease or an imbalance in nutrient intake. A CN looks closely at an individual's biochemical needs, physical activity levels, medication, nutrient depletion, lifestyle choices, and current nutrient intake to determine a course of action for that individual. A reputable CN will have a master's degree or PhD in human nutrition from an accredited university. Currently, there is no national certification or registration for CNs, so you will have to ask some questions to make sure you find a qualified practitioner.

You can ask your doctor for a recommendation, or look in your local phone book under "Nutrition" or "Dietician." Interview the practitioner in person or on the phone to get a sense of how he or she works. Find out where the CN got his or her education and what degrees and certifications he or she holds. Be suspicious of anyone who wants to sell you a lot of vitamins, supplements, or other products. You want someone who is primarily interested in helping you with your food intake.

Books

If you want to learn more about nutrition, *Eat, Drink, and Be Healthy: The Harvard Medical School Guide to Healthy Eating* by Walter C. Willett, MD, provides a fad-free approach to nutrition that is grounded in science and common sense. This book also contains over sixty pages of healthy and delicious recipes.

If you're interested in adopting a healthy approach to weight loss and eating well, I recommend the *Mayo Clinic Healthy Weight for Everybody* by Donald D. Hensrud, MD. For delicious and healthy recipes, I recommend *The New Mayo Clinic Cookbook: Eating Well for Better Health* by Donald Hensrud, MD.

Web Sites

For more information on nutrition, check out The Nutrition Source, a Web site maintained by the Harvard University School of Public Health: www.hsph.harvard.edu/nutritionsource.

You can find useful information on vitamins, minerals, supplements, and a host of health-related issues at www.wholehealthmd.com and www.medlineplus.gov. Another good Web site for researching supplements is www.herbmed.org. The University of Maryland's Center for Integrative Medicine posts valuable information on supplements at www.umm.edu/altmed/index.html.

The National Institutes of Health Office of Dietary Supplements provides helpful advice and good information on dietary supplements at dietary-supplements.info.nih.gov.

If you want to learn more about the glycemic index, visit www.glycemicindex.com.

Chapter 9: An Exercise Program That *Helps* More Than It *Hurts*

Videos

The Oregon Fibromyalgia Foundation offers several exercise videos for fibromyalgia patients. You can order them online at www.myalgia.com/Videos/Video_Introduction.htm.

The Arthritis Foundation offers exercise videos that are easy on the joints, including one on pool-based exercises. You can buy them online at www.arthritis.org.

The Integrative Movement Clinic offers exercise and relaxation videos designed for people with fibromyalgia and other painful conditions. You can find them at www.fibromyalgia-exercise-video.com.

The American Yoga Association Web site offers yoga videos and books for beginners at www.americanyoga association.org.

Web Sites

You can keep an online walking journal at www.in-motion.ca.

Chapter 10: A New Type of Drug for Fibromyalgia

You can research different medications to get information about benefits, side effects, and harmful interactions at www.medlineplus.gov.

Chapter 11: Complementary Therapies

The National Center for Complementary and Alternative Medicine provides comprehensive information on all types of complementary techniques at www.nccam.nih.gov. You can learn about the risks, benefits, and supporting evidence for the use of everything from acupuncture to tai chi.

Chapter 12: Moving Beyond Fibromyalgia

Support

Stay in touch with other people on the road to recovery. Join The Forum, an online support group, at www.drdryland. com.

A partial listing of fibromyalgia support groups by state is available at www.fmaware.org.

Job Accommodations

For more information on accommodations you may be entitled to in the workplace, visit the Job Accommodation Network's Web site at www.jan.wvu.edu/media/Fibro.html.

Recipe Ideas

Some recipes have ingredients in parentheses. You can safely add these ingredients as allowed in the challenge phase of the elimination protocol. If you are eliminating garlic, onions, tomatoes, and bell peppers (as recommended for IBS) during the elimination phase, you will need to modify these recipes.

Easy Guacamole (serves 4)

2 ripe avocados, peeled and pitted
(juice of ½ lime)
2 cloves garlic, minced
2 tbsp salsa (see recipe)
salt, to taste
1 tbsp fresh cilantro, chopped (optional)

In a small mixing bowl, mash the avocado with the (lime juice and) garlic. Stir in the salsa at the end, and adjust salt to taste. Add cilantro and stir, or sprinkle on top as a garnish.

Simple Salsa (serves 4)

1 tbsp olive oil
1 jalapeño pepper, seeded and minced (more, if you like it hotter)
½ small onion, finely chopped

1 to 3 cloves fresh garlic, minced
1 can Muir Glen roasted chopped tomatoes, or 4 to 6 fresh,
  organic, vine-ripened tomatoes of any kind, chopped
2 tbsp fresh cilantro, chopped
kosher or sea salt, to taste
(ground black pepper, to taste)

This dish can be served either warm or cold. For the cold version, combine all ingredients, except the olive oil, and refrigerate overnight so the flavors blend.

For the warm version, heat the olive oil in a 3-quart saucepan on low-medium heat. Add jalapeño, onions, and garlic and sauté for about 1 minute, stirring constantly. (Put the exhaust fan on! Heating peppers will cause them to release some of their volatile oils into the air and can start you coughing.) Turn the heat to low, and add the tomatoes carefully. (If the pan is very hot, they will splatter.) You may need to add a little water. Simmer for about 5 minutes. In the last minute, add the cilantro, and adjust the salt and pepper, to taste.

Olive and Artichoke Tapenade (serves 4–6)

1 can organic black olives
1 small can organic artichoke hearts in water
2 tbsp organic olive oil
1 sprig fresh rosemary
5 fresh sage leaves
1 tsp fresh thyme leaves
(ground black pepper, to taste)

Put all ingredients in food processor and chop until minced. Taste and adjust ingredients. Serve with celery sticks or jicama slices, or use as a stuffing for meats (during the challenge phase, fresh minced garlic can be added if you have no reaction).

Hummus *(serves 4–6)*

    1 cup dried garbanzo beans soaked overnight, rinsed, and simmered with a bay leaf until tender, or 1 large can garbanzo beans, drained and rinsed

    3 cloves garlic, peeled

    3 scallions with greens, chopped

    (juice of 1 Meyer lemon [can add a little grated rind as well])

    generous ¼ cup tahini

    1 tbsp olive oil and a little extra salt (or 2 tbsp tamari)

    1 tbsp cider vinegar

    ¼ tsp ground cumin

    ¼ tsp ground coriander

    ¼ tsp ground ginger

    ¼ tsp turmeric

    ½ tsp kosher salt

Put all ingredients in food processor and let it run until the consistency is what you want. Adjust spices to your taste. (You may want to add a little more salt.) Serve with vegetables or chips for dipping, or use as a sandwich spread.

All-Day Chili *(serves 3–4)*

Basic Ingredients:

    3 cups beans (kidney, black, red, pinto, anasazi—whichever you like or a blend)

    Best for your health: dried beans. Soak overnight in water with a dash of salt, rinse, and cook with a bay leaf in water on low-medium heat until tender.

Best for convenience: organic canned beans, rinsed
3 to 5 cloves garlic, minced
1 small yellow onion, chopped
1 can Muir Glen roasted tomatoes, crushed or chopped, or
   fresh tomatoes with about 2 cups of water
1 heaping tbsp ground cumin
1 heaping tbsp oregano
(2 heaping tbsp chili powder)
salt, to taste
(ground black pepper, to taste)
fresh cilantro, to taste

Options:

Vegetables—add whichever veggies you like: zucchini, summer squash, bell peppers, celery, corn, carrots, additional
hot green peppers (jalapeño, roasted chilies, poblanos,
habaneros, etc.) Meats—browned lean ground turkey or
chicken, or shredded chicken.

If you like your onions a little less pungent, sauté them with
the meat before adding them to the pot. In the morning,
put all ingredients in a slow cooker set to low. When you
get home, taste, adjust seasonings, and serve over a small
amount of rice with cilantro on top. (Add a sprinkling of
grated cheese on top during the challenge phase if you have
no reaction to dairy.)

Basic Salad Dressing

1 tsp Dijon-type mustard, smooth or grainy
2 tbsp + 1 tsp red wine vinegar or cider vinegar
½ cup extra virgin olive oil
1 tbsp expeller-pressed flaxseed oil

Whisk all ingredients together until combined.

Traditional Chicken Vegetable Soup (serves 3–4)

Stock:
   3 quarts water
   3 stalks celery, chopped coarsely
   3 carrots, chopped coarsely
   ½ yellow onion, chopped coarsely
   1 whole organic chicken, skinned, defatted, and cut up (leave bones in but not giblets)

Combine all ingredients and bring to a boil. Simmer, covered, for about one hour, or until chicken starts to fall off the bone. Remove the chicken and set aside, but leave the bones in the stock and continue to simmer, uncovered, until stock is reduced to your liking. Periodically skim and then strain the stock.

Soup:
   2 cloves garlic, minced
   ½ yellow onion, diced
   1 tsp olive oil
   2 quarts chicken stock
   2 carrots, diced
   2 stalks celery, diced
   1 cup sliced green beans—fresh if you can; frozen is second best
   meat from the chicken used to make the stock, chopped or shredded
   sea or kosher salt, to taste
   (freshly ground black pepper, to taste)
   tarragon or thyme or cilantro, to taste—fresh is best
   (1 cup corn—fresh if you can; frozen is second best)

Sauté garlic and onion in olive oil in the bottom of a large pot until onion is clear. Add stock, carrots, and celery, and bring to a boil. Lower heat to medium-low, and cook until carrots are just starting to get tender. Add green beans, chicken, and spices, and cook another 3 to 4 minutes. (Add corn about 1 minute before serving.) Adjust seasoning.

Optional additions:

chopped sweet potatoes: Add bite-size cubes about 3 minutes before carrots and celery.

broccoli: Steam separately, and add only to soup that will be served immediately and not stored.

green chilies: If canned, chop and add with green beans; if fresh, blanch or roast first.

Roasted Green Chili, White Bean, and Chicken Soup (serves 3–4)

- 2 tbsp organic olive oil (or 1½ tbsp olive oil and ½ tbsp hot pepper oil)
- 2 organic chicken breasts, skinned, boned, and diced
- 2 tsp Cajun seasoning
- 2 large, fresh, organic green chilies
- 1 medium organic leek, cut lengthwise and thinly sliced
- 2 cloves organic garlic, minced
- 2 quarts chicken broth—see above, but organic, free-range, store-bought is acceptable
- 2 cans organic cannellini beans or navy beans, or 1½ cups dried beans soaked overnight, rinsed, and simmered with a bay leaf until tender
- 2 tsp ground sea salt
- 2 tbsp fresh organic cilantro, chopped

In a large saucepan, heat oil on medium heat. Add diced chicken and Cajun seasoning. Sauté until nearly cooked through. Place chilies on a cookie sheet under the broiler. As the skin on the chilies bubbles and browns, turn so as much of the skin as possible is roasted. Remove from oven and let sit for about 5 minutes to cool. (The chilies will continue to steam inside their skins.) Add leek and garlic to the chicken mixture, and sauté until leeks become somewhat limp. When cool enough to handle, slice the tops off the chilies and split them lengthwise. Cut out the seeds and interior ridges, and peel the skin off the outsides. Dice the chilies, and add them to the chicken mixture. Add the remaining ingredients except the cilantro, and bring to a boil. Turn down heat and simmer for 20 minutes. In the last 5 minutes, add chopped cilantro. Adjust seasoning to taste, and serve with a fresh cilantro sprig as a garnish.

Purple Cabbage Salad (serves 1)

1 cup cabbage, shredded
¼ cup carrots, grated
¼ cup jicama, grated
1 tbsp pine nuts, lightly toasted
2 tbsp olive oil
2 tsp cider vinegar (or juice of ½ lime)
salt (and ground pepper), to taste

Mix all ingredients together in large bowl, and serve.

Informed Consent Form for Mirapex or Requip

This is the consent form I use with patients who are going to be taking either Mirapex or Requip. As we discussed in chapter 10, the use of these drugs for the treatment of fibromyalgia is a new and experimental treatment. This consent form ensures that patients understand the potential side effects of these medications when taken for fibromyalgia. If your doctor decides to follow the protocol described in chapter 10, you may need to sign something similar.

Informed Consent for the Administration of Medication

On _____ I had a conversation with Dr. _____
and he/she discussed the issues of this document:
I understand that my doctor, in diagnosing my condition, has included fibromyalgia. As part of my treatment, Dr. _____ has recommended I be given the following medication(s): Mirapex and/or Requip

1. Treatment Alternatives: The treatment alternatives include: analgesics, nonsteroidal anti-inflammatory agents, sleeping medications, muscle relaxants, and/or antidepressants.

2. Risks: This authorization is given with the understanding that any treatment involves some risks and hazards. I understand that it is not possible to anticipate all side effects.

   Some significant and substantial risks of this particular treatment were discussed earlier, with emphasis on sleepiness, nausea, gastrointestinal distress, anxiety, tremor, worsening sleep, vivid dreams, confusion, hallucinations, light-headedness, hair loss, agitation, fluid retention, and tremulousness. I was also informed that the use of Mirapex and/or Requip for fibromyalgia is not approved by the Food and Drug Administration. Its use for the treatment of fibromyalgia is considered experimental and off-label. I also have had it explained that some possible unknown side effects could occur when the drug is used at high doses for conditions other than Parkinson's disease.

3. Special Instructions: As a result of some of the potential side effects, I have been advised not to operate a motor vehicle or heavy machinery if I am sleepy or confused. Even if I am not sleepy or confused, I should still make a special effort to drive a vehicle only with extreme caution.

4. Gambling and other compulsive behaviors are potential side effects.

5. Pregnancy should be avoided while receiving the above medication.

6. Tagamet (cimetidine) should not be used in conjunction with Mirapex.

7. Cipro (ciprofloxacin) should not be used in conjunction with Requip. Other medications can interact with

Requip, and I will always discuss all medications used with Dr. _____.

IF YOU HAVE ANY QUESTIONS AS TO THE RISKS OR HAZARDS OF THE PROPOSED TREATMENT, OR ANY QUESTIONS CONCERNING THE PROPOSED TREATMENT, ASK YOUR PHYSICIAN NOW BEFORE SIGNING THIS CONSENT FORM!

DO NOT SIGN UNLESS YOU HAVE READ AND THOROUGHLY UNDERSTAND THIS FORM!

PATIENT'S CONSENT: I have read and fully understand this consent form. I understand I should not sign this form if treatment alternatives, risks, and special instructions have not been explained to my satisfaction. I further understand that I should not sign this form if I have unanswered questions or if I do not understand any of the terms or words used in this consent form. I give my consent to the administration of the above-named medications.

If I decide to stop taking the medications, I will contact my physician right away.

_____   _____
Patient/Responsible Party   Date

_____   _____
Witness   Date

8. PHYSICIAN DECLARATION: I have explained the contents of this document to the patient and have answered all the patient's questions, and to the best of my knowledge, I feel the patient has been adequately informed and has consented.

_____   _____
Physician's Signature   Date

Selected Bibliography

Chapter 1: The Frustration of Fibromyalgia

Croft, P., A.S. Rigby, R. Boswell, et al. "The Prevalence of Chronic Widespread Pain in the General Population." *Journal of Rheumatology.* 1993 Apr; 20(4):710–3.

Gremillion, R.B. "Fibromyalgia: Recognizing and Treating an Elusive Syndrome." *The Physician and Sportsmedicine.* 1998 Apr; 26(4):55–65.

National Institute of Arthritis and Musculoskeletal and Skin Diseases. National Institutes of Health. *Questions and Answers About Fibromyalgia.* June 2004.

Silverman, S., J. Mason. "Measuring the Functional Impact of FMS." *Journal of Musculoskeletal Medicine.* 1992; 9(7):15–24.

White, K.P., W.R. Nielson, M. Harth, et al. "Does the Label 'Fibromyalgia' Alter Health Status, Function, and Health Service Utilization?" *Arthritis and Rheumatism.* 2003 Feb 15; 49(1):144.

Wolfe F., J. Anderson, D. Harkness, et al. "A Prospective, Longitudinal, Multicenter Study of Service Utilization and Costs in Fibromyalgia." *Arthritis and Rheumatism.* 1997 Sep; 40(9):1560–70.

Wolfe, F., J. Anderson, D. Harkness, et al. "Work and Disability Status of Persons with Fibromyalgia." *Journal of Rheumatology.* 1997 Jun; 24(6):1171–8.

Wolfe, F., H.A. Smythe, M.B. Yunnus, et al. "The American College of Rheumatology 1990 Criteria for the Classification of Fibromyalgia." *Arthritis and Rheumatism.* 1990; 33(2):160–172.

Chapter 2: Making Sense of Fibromyalgia

Altier, N., J. Stewart. "The Role of Dopamine in the Nucleus Accumbens in Analgesia." *Life Sciences.* 1999; 65:2269–87.

Cohen, H., L. Neumann, A. Alhosshle, et al. "Abnormal Sympathovagal Balance in Men with Fibromyalgia." *Journal of Rheumatology.* 2001; 28:581–9.

Gambarana, C., F. Masi, A. Tagliamonte, et al. "A Chronic Stress That Impairs Reactivity in Rats Also Decreases Dopaminergic Transmission in the Nucleus Accumbens: A Microdialysis Study." *Journal of Neurochemistry.* 1999; 72:2039–46.

Holman, A. "Safety and Efficacy of the Dopamine Agonist Pramipexole on Pain Score for Refractory Fibromyalgia." *Arthritis and Rheumatism.* 2000; 43 (Supplement):S333.

Holman, H.J., R.R. Myers. "A Randomized, Double-Blind, Placebo-Controlled Trial of Pramipexole, a Dopamine Agonist, in Patients with Fibromyalgia Receiving Concomitant Medications." *Arthritis and Rheumatism.* 2005 Aug; 52(8):2495–505.

Martinez-Lavin, M., A. Hermosillo, M. Rosas, M. Soto. "Circadian Studies of Autonomic Nervous Balance in Patients with Fibromyalgia." *Arthritis and Rheumatism.* 1998; 41:1966–71.

Mountz, J., L. Bradley, G. Alarco. "Abnormal Functional Activity of the Central Nervous System in Fibromyalgia Syndrome." *American Journal of Medical Sciences* 1998; 315:385–96.

Quintero, L., M. Moreno, C. Avila, et al. "Long-Lasting Delayed Hyperalgesia After Subchronic Swim Stress." *Pharmacology, Biochemistry and Behavior.* 2000; 67:449–58.

Raj, S., D. Brouillard, C. Simpson, et al. "Dysautonomia Among Patients with Fibromyalgia: A Noninvasive Assessment." *Journal of Rheumatology.* 2000; 27:2660–5.

Routtinen, H., M. Partinen, C. Hublin, et al. "An FDOPA PET Study in Patients with Periodic Limb Movement Disorder and Restless Legs Syndrome." *Neurology.* 2000; 54:502–4.

Simms, R., S. Roy, M. Hrovat, et al. "Lack of Association Between Fibromyalgia Syndrome and Abnormalities in Muscle Energy Metabolism." *Arthritis and Rheumatism.* 1994; 37:794–800.

Snow, A., S. Tucker, W. Dewey. "The Role of Neurotransmitters in Stress-Induced Antinociception." *Pharmacology, Biochemistry and Behavior.* 1982; 16:47–50.

Torres, I., S. Cucco, M. Bassani, et al. "Long-Lasting Hyperalgesia After Chronic Restraint Stress in Rats—Effect of Morphine Administration." *Neuroscience Research.* 2003; 45:277–83.

Turjanski, N., A. Lees, D. Brooks. "Striatal Dopaminergic Function in Restless Legs Syndrome." *Neurology.* 1999; 52:932–7.

Vaeroy, H., Z. Qiao, L. Morkrid, et al. "Altered Sympathetic Nervous System Response in Patients with Fibromyalgia." *Journal of Rheumatology.* 1989; 16:1460–5.

Yunnus, M., J. Aldag. "Restless Legs Syndrome and Leg Cramps in Fibromyalgia Syndrome: A Controlled Study." *British Medical Journal.* 1996; 312:1339.

Yunnus M., A.T. Masi, J.J. Calabro, et al. "Primary Fibromyalgia (Fibrositis): Clinical Study of 50 Patients with Matched Normal Controls." *Seminars in Arthritis and Rheumatism.* 1981 Aug; 11(1):151–71.

Chapter 3: Understanding the Cause

Affleck, G., S. Urrow, H. Tennen, et al. "Sequential Daily Relations of Sleep, Pain Intensity, and Attention to Pain Among Women with Fibromyalgia." *Journal of Pain.* 1996; 68:363–8.

Davis, J., L. Loh, J. Nodal, et al. "Effects of Sleep on the Pattern of CO_2 Stimulated Breathing in Males and Females." *Proceedings of the Symposium on Regulation of Respiration During Sleep and Anesthesia* held at the Faculté de Médecine Saint-Antoine, Paris, France, July 14–16, 1977.

May, K., S. West, M. Baker, D. Everett. "Sleep Apnea in Male Patients with the Fibromyalgia Syndrome." *The American Journal of Medicine*. 1993; 94:505–8.

Moldofsky, H., P. Scarisbrick. "Induction of Neurasthenic Musculoskeletal Pain Syndrome by Selective Sleep State Deprivation." *Psychosomatic Medicine*. 1976 Jan–Feb; 38(1):35–44.

Ofluglu, D., O.H. Gunduz, E. Kul-Panza, Z. Guven. "Hypermobility in Women with Fibromyalgia Syndrome." *Clinical Rheumatology*. 2005 Oct 16; 1–3.

Pellegrino, M. "Atypical Chest Pain as an Initial Presentation of Primary Fibromyalgia." *Archives of Physical Medicine & Rehabilitation*. 1990; 71:526–8.

Taylor, S., L. Klein, B. Lewis, et al. "Biobehavioral Responses to Stress in Females: Tend-and-Befriend, Not Fight-or-Flight." *Psychological Review*. 2000; 107:411–9.

Chapter 4: Fibromyalgia and Other Conditions

Bennett, R. "Adult Growth Hormone Deficiency in Patients with Fibromyalgia." *Current Rheumatology Reports*. 2002; 4:306–12.

Park, D.C., J.M. Glass, M. Minear, et al. "Cognitive Function in Fibromyalgia Patients." *Arthritis and Rheumatism*. 2001 Sep; 44(9)2125–33.

Russell, I.J., M.D. Orr, B. Littman, et. al. "Elevated Cerebrospinal Fluid Levels of Substance P in Patients with the Fibromyalgia Syndrome." *Arthritis and Rheumatism*. 1994 Nov; 37(11):1593–601.

Veale, D., G. Kavanagh, J.F. Fielding, et al. "Primary Fibromyalgia and the Irritable Bowel Syndrome: Different Expressions of a Common Pathogenetic Process." *British Journal of Rheumatology*. 1991 Jun; 30(3):220–2.

Chapter 5: Do I Have Fibromyalgia?

Crofford, L.J., D.J. Clauw. "Fibromyalgia: Where Are We a Decade After the American College of Rheumatology Classification

Criteria Were Developed?" *Arthritis and Rheumatism.* 2002 May; 46 (5):1136–8.

Wolfe, F., H.A. Smythe, M.B. Yunnus, et al. "The American College of Rheumatology 1990 Criteria for the Classification of Fibromyalgia." Report of the Multicenter Criteria Committee. *Arthritis and Rheumatism.* 1990 Feb; 33(2):160–72.

Chapter 6: Sleeping Well

Affleck, G., S. Urrow, H. Tennen, et al. "Sequential Daily Relations of Sleep, Pain Intensity, and Attention to Pain Among Women with Fibromyalgia." *Journal of Pain.* 1996; 68:363–8.

Edinger, J., W.K. Wohlgemuth, A.D. Krystal, J.R. Rice. "Behavioral Insomnia Therapy for Fibromyalgia Patients: A Randomized Clinical Trial." *Archives of Internal Medicine.* 2005; 165:2527–35.

Jacobs, G. *Say Good Night to Insomnia.* New York: Henry Holt and Company, LLC. 1998.

Jacobs, G.D., E.F. Pace-Schott, R. Stickgold, M.W. Otto. "Cognitive Behavior Therapy and Pharmacotherapy for Insomnia: A Randomized Controlled Trial and Direct Comparison." *Archives of Internal Medicine.* 2004; 164:1888–96.

Moldofsky, H. "Sleep and Pain." *Sleep Medical Review.* 2001 Oct; 5(5):385–96.

Moldofsky, H., P. Scarisbrick. "Induction of Neurasthenic Musculoskeletal Pain Syndrome by Selective Sleep State Deprivation." *Psychosomatic Medicine.* 1976 Jan–Feb; 38(1):35–44.

Morin, C.M., M. Colecchi, J. Stone, et al. "Behavioral and Pharmacological Therapies for Late-Life Insomnia: A Randomized Controlled Trial." *Journal of the American Medical Association.* 1999; 281:991–9.

National Center on Sleep Disorder Research. National Heart, Lung, and Blood Institute. National Institutes of Health. *Insomnia: Assessment and Management in Primary Care.* September, 1998.

National Institute of Neurological Disorders and Stroke. National Institutes of Health. *Brain Basics: Understanding Sleep.* Available at www.ninds.nih.gov.

National Sleep Foundation. *2002 Sleep in America Poll.* Available at www.sleepfoundation.org.

Ringdahl, E., S. Pereira, J.E. Delzell. "Treatment of Primary Insomnia." *Journal of the American Board of Family Practitioners.* 2004 May–June; 17 (3):212–9.

Roizenblatt, S., H. Moldofsky, A.A. Benedito-Silva, S. Tufik. "Alpha Sleep Characteristics in Fibromyalgia." *Arthritis and Rheumatism.* 2001 Jan; 44(1):222–30.

Smith, M., M. Perlis, A. Park, et al. "Comparative Meta-analysis of Pharmacotherapy and Behavior Therapy for Persistent Insomnia." *American Journal of Psychiatry.* 2002; 159: 5–11.

Wagner, J., M. Wagner, W. Hening. "Beyond Benzodiazepines: Alternative Pharmacologic Agents for the Treatment of Insomnia." *Annals of Pharmocotherapy.* 1998; 32:680–91.

Chapter 7: Reducing Stress: Easier Said Than Done

Aftanas, L., S. Golosheykin. "Impact of Regular Meditation Practice on EEG Activity at Rest and During Evoked Negative Emotions." *International Journal of Neuroscience.* 2005 Jun; 115(6):893–909.

Davidson, R.J., J. Kabat-Zinn, J. Schumacher, et al. "Alterations in Brain and Immune Function Produced by Mindfulness Meditation." *Psychosomatic Medicine.* 2003 Jul–Aug; 65(4):564–70.

Kaplan, K.H., D.L. Goldenberg, M. Galvin-Nadeau. "The Impact of a Meditation-Based Stress Reduction Program on Fibromyalgia." *General Hospital Psychiatry.* 1993 Sep; 15(5):284–9.

Lewis, T., F. Amini, R. Lannon. *A General Theory of Love.* New York: Random House. 2001.

Maclean, C.R., K.G. Walton, D.K. Levitsky, et al. "Effects of the Transcendental Meditation Program on Adaptive Mechanisms:

Changes in Hormone Levels and Response to Stress After four Months' Practice." *Psychoneuroendocrinology.* 1997 May; 22(4):277–95.

National Center for Complementary and Alternative Medicine. *Meditation for Health Purposes.* Available at http://nccam. nih.gov/health/meditation/.

Rosenberg, M. *Nonviolent Communication: A Language of Life: Create Your Life, Your Relationships, and Your World in Harmony with Your Values* (2nd edition). California: Puddle-dancer Press. 2003.

Chapter 8: Eating Well and Feeling Better

Adler, G.K., B.T. Kinsley, S. Hurwitz, et al. "Reduced Hypothalamic-Pituitary and Sympathoadrenal Responses to Hypoglycemia in Women with Fibromyalgia Syndrome." *The American Journal of Medicine.* 1999 May; 106(5):534–43.

Bagis, S., L. Tamer, G. Sahin. "Free Radicals and Antioxidants in Primary Fibromyalgia: An Oxidative Stress Disorder?" *Rheumatology International.* 2005 Apr; 25(3):188–90.

Caruso, I., P. Sarzi-Puttini, M. Cazzola, et al. "Double-Blind Study of 5-hydroxy-L-tryptophan Versus Placebo in the Treatment of Primary Fibromyalgia Syndrome." *Journal of International Medical Research.* 1990 May–Jun; 18(3):201–9.

Choi, H.K. "Dietary Risk Factors for Rheumatic Diseases." *Current Opinion Rheumatology.* 2005 Mar; 17(2):141–6.

Donaldson, M., N. Speight, S. Loomis. "Fibromyalgia Syndrome Improved Using a Mostly Raw Vegetarian Diet: An Observational Study." *BMC Complementary and Alternative Medicine.* 2001:7.

Fava, M., J. Alpert, A.A. Nierenberg, et al. "A Double-Blind, Randomized Trial of St. John's Wort, Fluoxetine, and Placebo in Major Depressive Disorder. *Journal of Clinical Psychopharmacology.* 2005 Oct; 25(5):441–7.

Foran, J.A., D.O. Carpenter, M.C. Hamilton, et al. "Risk-Based Consumption Advice for Farmed Atlantic and Wild Pacific

Salmon Contaminated with Dioxins and Dioxin-like Compounds. *Environmental Health Perspectives.* 2005 May; 113(5):552–6.

Graham, T.E., V. Sgro, D. Friars, M.J. Gibala. "Glutamate Ingestion: The Plasma and Muscle Free Amino Acid Pools of Resting Humans." *American Journal of Physiology, Endocrinology and Metabolism,* 2000; 278(1):E83–E89.

Herzallah, S.M., M.A. Humeid, K.M. Al-Ismail. "Effect of Heating and Processing Methods of Milk and Dairy Products on Conjugated Linoleic Acid and Trans Fatty Acid Isomer Content." *Journal of the American College of Nutrition.* 1994 Apr; 13(2):209–10.

Jacobsen, S., B. Danneskiold-Samsoe, R.B. Anderson. "Oral S-adenosylmethionine in Primary Fibromyalgia: Double-Blind Clinical Evaluation." *Scandinavian Journal of Rheumatology.* 1991; 20(4):294–302.

Kaartinen, K., K. Lammi, et al. "Vegan Diet Alleviates Fibromyalgia Symptoms." *Scandinavian Journal of Rheumatology.* 2000; 29(5):308–13.

Kelly, G.S. "Nutritional and botanical interventions to assist with the adaptation to stress." *Alternative Medicine Review.* 1999 Aug; 4(4):249–65.

Kim, L.S., L.J. Axelrod, P. Howard, N. Buratovich, R.F. Waters. "Efficacy of Methylsulfonylmethane (MSM) in Osteoarthritis Pain of the Knee: A Pilot Clinical Trial." *Osteoarthritis Cartilage.* 2005 Nov 22; [Epub ahead of print]

McGinnis, J.M., W.H. Foege. "Actual Causes of Death in the United States." *Journal of the American Medical Association.* 1993; 270(18): 2207–12.

Minino, A., L. Smith. National Center for Health Statistics, Centers for Disease Control and Prevention, U.S. Department of Health and Human Services. "Deaths: Preliminary Data for 2000." *National Vital Statistics Report.* 2001; 49(12).

Ozgocmen, S., H. Ozyurt, S. Sogut, et al. "Antioxidant Status, Lipid Peroxidation Inaccurate Oxide in Fibromyalgia: Etiologic and Therapeutic Concerns." *Rheumatology International.* 2005 Nov 10; 1–6.

Puttini, P.S., I. Caruso. "Primary Fibromyalgia Syndrome and 5-hydroxy-L-tryptophan: A 90-day Open Study." *Journal of International Medical Research.* 1992 Apr; 20(2):182–9.

Russell, I.J., J.E. Michalek, J.D. Flechas, G.E. Abraham. "Treatment of Fibromyalgia Syndrome with Super Malic: A Randomized, Double-Blind, Placebo-Controlled, Crossover Pilot Study." *Journal of Rheumatology.* 1995 May; 22(5):953–8.

Smith, J.D., C.M. Terpening, S.O. Schmidt, et al. "Relief of Fibromyalgia Symptoms Following Discontinuation of Dietary Excitotoxins. *Annals of Pharmacotherapy.* 2001 Jun; 35(6): 702–6.

Steinman, David. *Diet for a Poisoned Planet.* New York: Ballantine Books. 1992.

Wintergerst, E.S., S. Maggini, D.H. Hornig. "Immune-Enhancing Role of Vitamin C and Zinc and Effect on Clinical Conditions." *Annals of Nutrition and Metabolism.* 2005 Dec 21; 50(2):85–94. [Epub ahead of print]

Chapter 9: An Exercise Program That *Helps* More Than It *Hurts*

Altan, L., U. Bingol, M. Aykae, Z. Koe, M. Yurtkuran. "Investigation of the Effects of Pool-Based Exercise on Fibromyalgia Syndrome." *Rheumatology International.* 2004 Sep; 24(5):272–7.

Da Costa, D., M. Abrahamowicz, I. Lowensteyn, et al. "A Randomized Clinical Trial of an Individualized Home-Based Exercise Program for Women with Fibromyalgia." *Rheumatology.* 2005 Nov; 44(11):1422–7.

DiBenedetto, M., K.E. Innes, A.G. Taylor, et al. "Effect of a Gentle Iyengar Yoga Program on Gait in the Elderly: An Exploratory Study." *Archives of Physical Medical Rehabilitation.* 2005 Sep; 86(9):1830–7.

Dobkin, P.L., M. Abrahamowicz, M.A. Fitzcharles, et al. "Maintenance of Exercise in Women with Fibromyalgia." *Arthritis and Rheumatism.* 2005 Oct 15; 53(5):724–31.

Dupree, J., S. Clark. "Individualizing the Exercise Prescription for Persons with Fibromyalgia." *Rheumatic Disease Clinics of North America.* 2002; 28:419–6.

Dupree, J., S. Clark, R. Bennett. "Prescribing Exercise for People with Fibromyalgia." *AACN Clinical Issues.* 2002; 13(2)277–93.

Dupree, J., S. Clark, C.S. Burckhard, et al. "Exercise for Patients with Fibromyalgia: Risks Versus Benefits." *Current Rheumatology Reports.* 2001; 3:135–40.

Gowans, S.E., A. Dehueck. "Effectiveness of Exercise in Management of Fibromyalgia." *Current Opinion Rheumatology.* 2004 Mar; 16(2):138–42.

Gowans, S.E., A. Dehueck, S. Voss, A. Silaj, S.E. Abbey. "Six-Month and One-Year Follow-Up of 23 Weeks of Aerobic Exercise for Individuals with Fibromyalgia." *Arthritis and Rheumatism.* 2004 Dec 15; 51(6):890–8.

Jentoft, E.S., A.G. Kvalvik, A.M. Mengshoel. "Effects of Pool-Based and Land-Based Aerobic Exercise on Women with Fibromyalgia/Chronic Widespread Muscle Pain." *Arthritis and Rheumatism.* 2001 Feb; 45(1):42–7.

Jones, K.D., C.S. Burckhardt, S.R. Clark, R.M. Bennett, K.M. Potempa. "A Randomized Controlled Trial of Muscle Strengthening Versus Flexibility Training in Fibromyalgia." *Journal of Rheumatology.* 2002 May; 29(5):1041–8.

Kingsley, J.D., L.B. Panton, T. Toole, et al. "The Effects of a 12-Week Strength-Training Program on Strength and Functionality in Fibromyalgia." *Archives of Physical Medical Rehabilitation.* 2005 Sep; 86(9):1713–21.

Mannerkorpi, K. "Exercise in Fibromyalgia." *Current Opinion Rheumatology.* 2005 Mar; 17(2):190–4.

Mannerkorpi, K., B. Nyberg, M. Ahlmen, C. Ekdahl. "Pool Exercise Combined with an Education Program for Patients with Fibromyalgia Syndrome." *Journal of Rheumatology.* 2000 Oct; 27(10):2473–81.

Meiworm, L., E. Jakob, U.A. Walter, et al. "Patients with Fibromyalgia Benefit from Aerobic Endurance Exercise." *Clinical Rheumatology.* 2000; 19(4):253–7.

Mengshoel, A.M., H.B. Komnaes, O. Forre. "The Effects of 20 Weeks of Physical Fitness Training in Female Patients with Fibromyalgia." *Clinical Experimental Rheumatology.* 1992 Jul–Aug; 10(4):345–9.

Meyer, B.B., K.J. Lemley. "Utilizing Exercise to Affect the Symptomology of Fibromyalgia: A Pilot Study." *Med. Science Sports Exercise.* 2000 Oct; 32(10):1691–7.

Michalsen, A., P. Grossman, A. Acil, et al. "Rapid Stress Reduction and Anxiolysis Among Distressed Women as a Consequence of a Three-Month Intensive Yoga Program." *Medical Science Monitor.* 2005 Nov 24; 11(12):CR555–61.

Pilkington, K., G. Kirkwood, H. Rampes, J. Richardson. "Yoga for Depression: The Research Evidence." *Journal of Affective Disorders.* 2005 Dec; 89(1–3):13–24.

Sherman, K.J., D.C. Cherkin, J. Erro, et al. "Comparing Yoga, Exercise, and a Self-Care Book for Chronic Low Back Pain: A Randomized Controlled Trial." *Annals of Internal Medicine.* 2005; 143:849–56.

Sim, J., N. Adams. "Systematic Review of Randomized Controlled Trials of Nonpharmacological Interventions for Fibromyalgia." *The Clinical Journal of Pain.* 2002; 18:324–36.

Song, R., E.O. Lee, P. Lam, S.C. Bae. "Effects of Tai Chi Exercise on Pain, Balance, Muscle Strength, and Perceived Difficulties in Physical Functioning in Older Women with Osteoarthritis." *Journal of Rheumatology.* 2003 Sep; 30(9):2039–44.

Taggart, H.M., C.L. Arslanian, S. Bae, K. Singh. "Effects of T'ai Chi Exercise on Fibromyalgia Symptoms and Health-Related Quality of Life." *Orthopedic Nursing.* 2003 Sep–Oct; 22(5):353–60.

Chapter 10: A New Type of Drug for Fibromyalgia

Holman, H.J., R.R. Myers. "A Randomized, Double-Blind, Placebo-Controlled Trial of Pramipexole, a Dopamine Agonist, in Patients with Fibromyalgia Receiving Concomitant Medications." *Arthritis and Rheumatism.* 2005 Aug; 52(8):2495–505.

Yunnus, M.B., A.T. Masi, J.C. Aldag. "Short-Term Effects of Ibuprofen in Primary Fibromyalgia Syndrome: A Double-Blind, Placebo-Controlled Trial." *Journal of Rheumatology.* 1989 Apr; 16(4):527–32.

Chapter 11: Complementary Therapies

"Acupuncture Relieves Symptoms of Fibromyalgia, Mayo Clinic Study Finds." *Medical News Today.* August 26, 2005. Available at www.medicalnewstoday.com.

Alvarez, D.J., P.G. Rockwell. "Trigger Points: Diagnosis and Management." *American Family Physician.* 2002; 65(4):653–60.

Assefi, N.P., K.J. Sherman, C. Jacobsen, et al. "A Randomized Clinical Trial of Acupuncture Compared with Sham Acupuncture in Fibromyalgia." *Annals of Internal Medicine.* 2005 Jul 5; 143(1):124.

Birch, S., J.K. Hesselink, F.A. Jonkman, et al. "Clinical Research on Acupuncture. Part 1. What Have Reviews of the Efficacy and Safety of Acupuncture Told Us So Far?" *Journal of Alternative and Complementary Medicine.* 2004 Jun; 10(3):468–80.

Blunt, K.L., M.H. Rajwani, R.C. Guerriero. "The Effectiveness of Chiropractic Management of Fibromyalgia Patients: A Pilot Study." *Journal of Manipulative Physiological Therapy.* 1997 Jul–Aug; 20(6):389–99.

Brattberg, G. "Connective Tissue Massage in the Treatment of Fibromyalgia." *European Journal of Pain.* 1999 Jun; 3(3):235–44.

Gamber, R.G., J.H. Shores, D.P. Russo, et al. "Osteopathic Manipulative Treatment in Conjunction with Medication Relieves Pain Associated with Fibromyalgia Syndrome: Results of a Randomized Clinical Pilot Project." *Journal of the American Osteopathic Association*. 2002 Jun; 102(6):321–5.

Hains, G., F. Hains. "A Combined Ischemic Compression and Spinal Manipulation in the Treatment of Fibromyalgia: A Preliminary Estimate of Dose and Efficacy." *Journal of Manipulative Physiological Therapy*. 2000 May; 23(4):225–30.

National Center for Complementary and Alternative Medicine. National Institutes of Health. *Get the Facts: Acupuncture*. December 2004. Available at http://nccam.nih.gov/health/.

Index

About the Authors

DAVID DRYLAND, MD, is a Yale-trained clinical rheumatologist with a busy practice in Medford, Oregon. Having successfully won his own battle with fibromyalgia, Dr. Dryland has developed a groundbreaking treatment protocol that his own patients have followed with success. A much sought-after speaker, Dr. Dryland leads seminars and workshops on how to recover from fibromyalgia and control the fight-or-flight response. He lives in Ashland, Oregon, with his wife Laurel and his three children.

LORIE LIST is a freelance writer living in Ashland, Oregon. Now fully recovered from fibromyalgia, she spends her free time hiking, riding horses, practicing yoga, and kayaking with her husband Jason.